CANCER
WASN'T ON MY BUCKET LIST!

A Personal Journal

BREE KAYSON

ILLUSTRATED BY DREW MESSINA

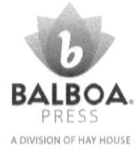

BALBOA.
PRESS

A DIVISION OF HAY HOUSE

Balboa Press books may be ordered through booksellers or by contacting:

Balboa Press
A Division of Hay House
1663 Liberty Drive
Bloomington, IN 47403
www.balboapress.com
1 (877) 407-4847

Print information available on the last page.

ISBN: 978-1-5043-6412-6 (sc)
ISBN: 978-1-5043-6411-9 (hc)
ISBN: 978-1-5043-6410-2 (e)

Library of Congress Control Number: 2016912953

Balboa Press rev. date: 11/03/2016

To My Amazing Husband, Son, and Daughter—
Thank you for giving me the freedom to over share.
I love you beyond measure.

My heart is full of gratitude for everyone who has taken this journey beside me.

Special thanks to:

Larry, this would still be on my list of things to do if not for you. Thank you for helping me to check this one off! I appreciate your honest reviews and the many hours you spent reading copy. Your never-ending support means the world to me.

Drew, thank you for demonstrating your outstanding artistic talent!

Lauren, thank you for lifting me up every step of the way!

Mikki, you were the first person to read my manuscript. Without your positive feedback this would not be in print.

Wanda and Bernie, where would I be without your loving guidance and support during those early years? I am eternally grateful for you both.

Ann, you are a beautiful soul! I will forever treasure the memories.

Bri, among other things, many thanks for making "that phone call" when I needed it. Somehow, you just know!

Charles, thank you for your compassionate insight and guidance.

My "breast friend" Kim, I am profoundly thankful for your ever-present support on this bumpy ride.

My amazing doctors, thank you for your patience with all my questions. I am thankful for your kindness, understanding, and your expertise.

For so many friends and family, I am blessed to have you in my life. I appreciate each and every one of you.

Contents

PART 1: FEEL TO HEAL 1

Chapter 1: Until Life Do Us Part 3

Chapter 2: Come Sail Away.......................................14

Chapter 3: Did I Sign Up for This? 23

Chapter 4: The Wonder of Waves 36

Chapter 5: Seventy Countries....................................44

PART 2: MY PERSONAL JOURNAL 51

Chapter 6: She Said Those Words: "It Is Cancer".....................53

Chapter 7: This Just Got Real: Waiting Rooms, Exam Rooms, and Operating Rooms 65

Chapter 8: What Are My Surgery Options? 84

Chapter 9: To Chemo or Not to Chemo? 101

Chapter 10: My Body Feels Toxic.............................122

Chapter 11: My New Normal....................................139

Chapter 12: Some Moments Change Us.....................151

PART ONE

Feel to Heal

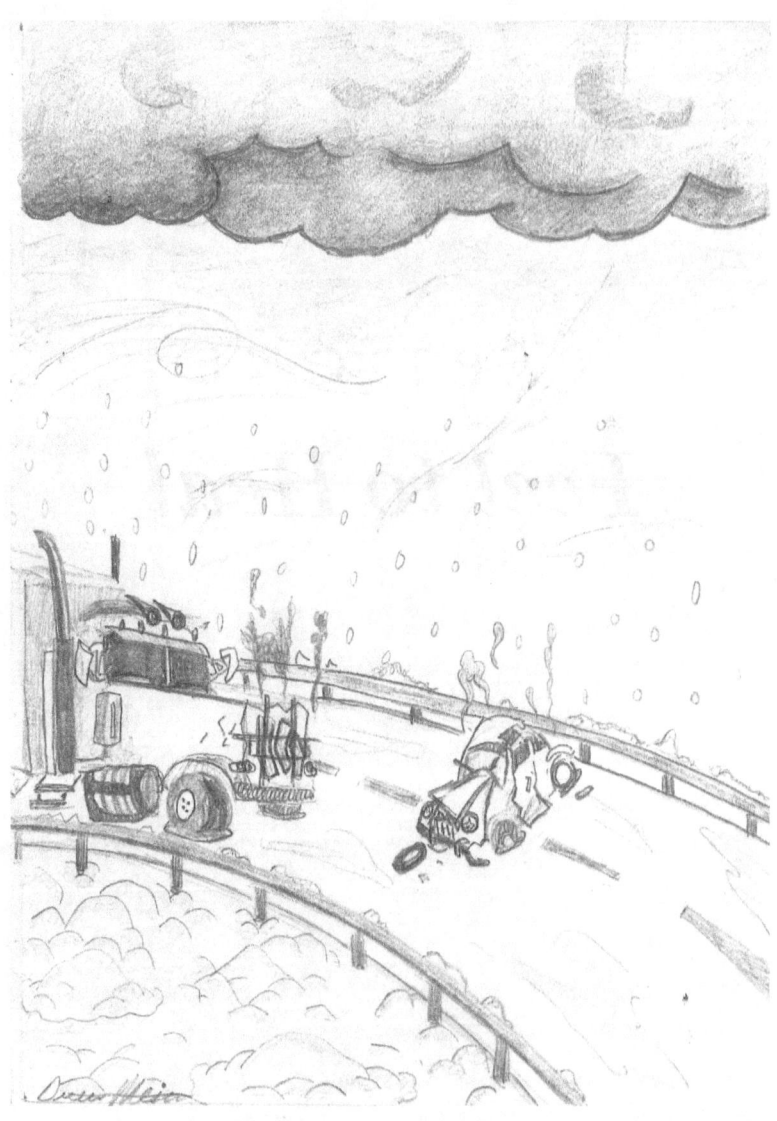

CHAPTER 1

Until Life Do Us Part

My mom died when I was thirteen. I wanted to die too.

It was dinnertime, and I was happy to be spending the night at my oldest brother's house. Despite our age difference of twenty-three years, Mike and I had a close bond. That winter night as we gathered together, my brother and sister-in-law took their places at either end of the oval table. My nine-year-old nephew plopped down in his usual chair, and I found my seat across the table from my gleeful sixteen-year-old niece.

In my family, it was customary to say grace before we ate a meal. From a teenager's perspective, these prayers always seemed longer than necessary. So while Mike recited the blessing, my niece and I playfully made a game of peaking through squinty eyes and trying not to giggle.

We had just filled our plates when suddenly the telephone started to ring, interrupting our festive conversation. My brother jumped up to answer the call. "Hello," I heard him say. Then there was a long pause before, "Okay. We'll be right there." When he returned to the table, the distressed look on his face told me something was wrong—very wrong.

"There has been a car accident," he said. "We need to go to the hospital." Leaving the table as it was, we all grabbed our coats and quickly piled into the freezing car.

3

During the silent drive to the hospital, I was scared and felt an overwhelming sense of dread. Tension filled the air. Deep down I knew this wasn't going to be good.

As soon as we walked into the stark hospital lobby, I was ushered into a small waiting area to sit with my niece and nephew. Somebody (I don't recall who) brought me my mom's purse for safekeeping; I looked inside and pulled out her glasses. They were broken and covered with blood. I remember holding them in my hand and thinking, *If this is what her glasses look like, what does she look like?* When I finally saw my brother walking down the hall toward me, his face was full of anguish. My breath stopped short, and my heart began to pound. I could see that he had been crying. Somehow he choked out the words that our mom was gone; she had perished. Suddenly I became dizzy. I collapsed, falling into his arms. The next thing I knew we were in the hospital chapel. I heard myself hysterically screaming, "No no no! God, please no! Not my mommy! Not my mommy!" I couldn't believe my mother was dead! She wouldn't be coming home. Not tonight. Not ever.

It was a horrific collision. Wintertime in Nebraska can be treacherous, and it had been snowing heavily. The roads were wet and icy. My dad, mom, sister, and two of her children had been on their way home from a funeral. As they approached an incline in the two-lane road, their car slid across into the oncoming traffic lane. At that moment, a semi-trailer truck came over the hill and slammed into the Volkswagen Bug full force. Everyone but my nephew was seriously injured. We were told that Mom died instantly. At the scene, my father was in shock and kept trying to wake her. He slapped her face repeatedly, begging her to open her eyes. I guess knowing she didn't suffer made us feel a little bit better.

The day before the accident, Mom had given me a choice. I could skip school and go to the funeral with them, or I could stay at my brother's house and he would take me to school the next morning. Surprisingly I chose school over taking the trip. Maybe going to a funeral didn't sound like much fun, or maybe I just wasn't supposed to be in that car.

When I think back on the evening before the accident, I wonder if my mom knew that her time was short. That night she abandoned her usual routine and stayed up late sorting papers, paying bills, and organizing things. Some people believe we subconsciously know when we've completed the lessons we came here to learn. Maybe we do.

The next three days were a blur. I remember lying on the sofa in a despondent state, hoping against hope that it was all just a bad dream. I would have done anything to bring her back, but I knew I couldn't. The day of the funeral came too soon and made her death all too real. The church was full of people, but I couldn't see faces. I was focused on the casket at the front of the church. At one point during my mom's favorite song, I was crying so loud that my dad switched seats so that I could be next to him. At the conclusion of the service, the casket was slowly escorted to the back of the church. It was then opened so that everyone could say their good-byes as they exited the sanctuary. As I moved toward her lifeless body, I suddenly threw my arms around her and sobbed, pleading with her not to leave me. I was shocked at how cold—freezing cold—she was. She hated being cold. Her soft and caring body was now hard and stiff. It hit me like a freight train...She would never play Yahtzee with me again. She would never sleep with me when I was scared. Someone—I don't remember who—had to pry me off of her.

I felt so damn cheated! One day I hated her for leaving me, and the next day I was begging God to bring her to back. I loved my dad too, but at thirteen my mom had been my world. The anguish was physically painful, and my very soul hurt.

Being the youngest of eight children, I was the only one still living at home when the accident happened. My father was a strong man, but he was going through his own agony. Often I would wake in the middle of the night and hear him scream out and cry in his sleep. He would relive the sights and sounds of the horrible crash over and over.

At sixty-three, my father was older than most parents of teenagers back then, and over the next couple of years I became quite a handful. I was angry and defiant. I didn't worry about consequences. I had survived losing my mom—what could be worse?

Adjusting to my new normal, I was excited to be starting high school with my new friend, Susan. We had met while attending a youth group at church and quickly became thick as thieves. Susan was tall and athletic. She had dark, wavy hair, and her brown eyes revealed a hint of sadness. In contrast, I was somewhat short and very thin. My blonde hair was stick straight, and my blue eyes were usually hidden behind glasses.

Susan was a risk taker and had a rebellious side. Our silly antics made me remember what it felt like to laugh. We planned sleepovers at each other's houses almost every weekend.

Then one winter afternoon we went snow tubing. The steep hill was a popular spot, and it was overcrowded that day. We finally found a space at the top of the hill and tried to fit both our bodies on one tube. Soon after we pushed off and gained speed, things went horribly wrong. Susan fell off and was run over by another flying snow tube.

Stopping the slippery tube as soon as I could, I rushed over to where she was lying on the snow. She could barely move. Someone called an ambulance. At the hospital, we learned that Susan had a serious back injury. She would eventually fully recover, but it would take a few months. I felt terrible; I was guilt-ridden that she had been hurt and I hadn't been injured. Apparently she resented me for the same reason. She became distant and hostile toward me. Things were never the same. Ultimately, unable to mend the friendship, we went our separate ways.

During my junior year, when I was sixteen, I was miserable and threatened to quit high school. I was insecure and low on self-esteem. This was mostly due to the fact that someone had been leaving me anonymous threatening notes. I was always looking over my shoulder wondering who it could be. Eventually I learned that "the someone" was my former best friend. It was easy for me to become paranoid when I didn't know the identity of my enemy, but finding out it was someone I had trusted so deeply was devastating.

Needing a fresh start and new surroundings, I called my sister Faye to ask if I could come live with her while I finished high school. She lived with her husband, Ben, and their three children in a town five hundred miles away.

Reluctantly, my father agreed to let me go. As I stepped up to board that daunting Greyhound bus, I looked back to mouth "I love you." I felt guilty for leaving him. He looked so sad. He was worried about me. As I settled into my seat, I was flooded with conflicting emotions. I needed this change, but I was abandoning my dad. He would now be living alone. Without warning, I felt angry with my mom. Her departure felt like a betrayal. One day she'd kissed me good night, and the next day—poof!—she was gone. The emotions of that excruciating day came rushing back. I was alone and empty inside.

Staring out that dirty bus window was cathartic. The little towns came and went. People came and went. Eventually, I fell asleep.

A few hours later, I awoke with a renewed sense of purpose. Even though moving to a new a new school was scary and somewhat intimidating, I was looking forward to the detour.

Faye and Ben welcomed me into their home and loved me unconditionally. Looking back, I realize that was quite the undertaking—adding a teenager to their household when they already had three young children.

I was happy to learn their babysitter attended the same high school where I was enrolling. She kindly offered to introduce me to some high school kids who lived in the neighborhood. There were about ten in the group. The babysitter and I didn't have much in common, but one of the other girls and I formed a quick bond. We both had adventurous spirits. Unfortunately, we sometimes channeled that into experimenting with drugs and alcohol. I knew I shouldn't get involved with those things, but I did anyway, trying everything from marijuana to mescaline and cocaine. We definitely kept our guardian angels busy!

I lost my virginity that summer. Let's just say the rondezvous wasn't quite what I had envisioned. I was under the impression he "really cared" about me. Pretty sure he doesn't remember my name.

There must have been times when my sister and her husband regretted taking in a reckless teenager, but they never once threatened to send me back home. I am eternally grateful to them, as I have no doubt my life would have taken a downward spiral without their influence and compassion.

During my senior year of high school, I met Greg. It was a Friday night; we were at the house party of a mutual friend. I noticed him standing in the small kitchen as I tried to open a bottle of wine. He sweetly asked, "Can I help you with that?" "Sure," I replied. "You're probably better at it than I am!" His thick blond hair was unruly and touched his shoulders. He skillfully opened the bottle and poured two glasses. We made our way out to the patio. I learned that Greg was three years older than I. He was engaging and had a quick smile. We had sudden chemistry. His quiet confidence made him sexy. Before that party ended, we had made plans to see each other again.

Our connection quickly evolved into a serious relationship. He was twenty-one, and I was just eighteen years old when we married. We were crazy in love, and no one could have stopped us!

Deliriously happy that first year, we were ecstatic to be moving into our new home. It was bigger than we needed, but we planned to have a family someday.

Greg was an auto mechanic. I enrolled in beauty school and graduated with a license in cosmetology. I had a passion for hairstyling, and I was good at it. Making people feel better about themselves made me feel good too.

Greg and I matured during the next few years; we grew up. Unfortunately, we also grew apart. I was unhappy and feeling disconnected. Maybe we married too young.

One afternoon at work, I met Brian. We developed a friendship that rapidly progressed into an extra-marital relationship. The intense guilt I felt did not stop me. I knew the affair was wrong. I just didn't care. How could I do this to Greg?

It wasn't a secret for long; Greg had suspicions and did some investigating. When he confronted me, I did not deny it. I felt terrible about the pain I was causing him. The marriage spiraled out of control. It didn't happen overnight, but the steady descent into emotional chaos gradually made my life feel like some sort of black hole.

Divorce was inevitable. We separated just before our fourth anniversary. It wasn't long before Brian started pressuring me to get married. It was overwhelming. I abruptly ended the relationship.

Why had I made such a mess of things? Greg had loved me unconditionally. Why hadn't that been enough? Was I trying to fill the emptiness that losing my mom had triggered? Was I afraid to fully love someone, for fear of losing him?

At the age of twenty-two, I wasn't sure about the future. Greg and I agreed that he could keep the house, and I would move out. I was fine with that. In fact, having my own place would be liberating. Hastily, I found a tiny apartment near the salon where I worked. This was great; I could do whatever I wanted, whenever I wanted!

Okay—it wasn't all that great. There were a lot of nights that saw me crying myself to sleep because I was lonely and scared.

The chic salon was prestigious and fast paced. I loved working there. However, it didn't take long to realize that I needed a second job in order to support myself. A posh new bar and restaurant was opening across the street from the salon; they were hiring servers and bartenders. Having zero experience waiting on tables and no clue about bartending, I applied anyway. To my surprise, I was offered a position, and they were willing to train me!

I felt lucky and thrilled to have the job; things were looking up. Then, just a few months later, we were notified that the restaurant wasn't doing well and would be closing soon. I immediately started applying at restaurants that had openings for servers. The gods were smiling on me—I was able to land a part-time server position in an upscale steakhouse.

During the summer of 1983, I met Tina, another server at the steakhouse. She was spontaneous and had a quirky sense of humor. Blessed with the body of a gymnast, she was athletically fit. Being a novice runner myself, I was impressed that Tina competed in marathons.

We both loved to run, and going out for a five-mile run after work at midnight wasn't unusual. We hit the gym regularly too. Conversely, we didn't hesitate to party. I remember blowing $300 in one night on cocaine—not that either one of us could afford that! Since Tina and I practically lived together anyway, we thought getting a place together would be a good idea. Splitting expenses would benefit both of us. We found a charming two-bedroom apartment not far from where we worked.

Having a roommate was great. We worked hard and played harder. We had some crazy times, including a night of group sex. I vaguely remember riding topless in a friend's Jaguar convertible, waving at everyone like we were in a parade. I blame the martinis!

Waiting tables was hard work, but the staff was a tight-knit group, and we managed to make it fun. Most days I actually looked forward to going to work, although anyone who has worked in the industry knows that the real party begins after hours when the restaurant closes.

Working in a restaurant provides opportunities to meet some interesting people. There was the undercover detective who would place his pistol on the nightstand when he slept over, sexy or creepy-I wasn't sure! Some said a mysterious bartender was involved with the mafia. All I know is he didn't like to linger in front of windows.

Going out dancing after work was always an adventure. At a trendy club one night, I befriended the strikingly handsome, news anchor of a local TV station. When we went to a restaurant, he had to sit facing the door; He liked to be recognized. And who could forget the Michael Jackson impersonator? I'm convinced he actually believed he was Michael Jackson.

Newly divorced, I felt free. Free to take risks. Free to make reckless decisions.

One magical day, after collecting my mail, I opened an envelope to find a pre-approved new credit card with my name on it. I couldn't believe my eyes; it felt like a gift from above. So what did I do? Drove straight to the mall and bought a fabulous pair of shoes! Justifiable, right? Within the week, Tina and I had decided we would take a Caribbean cruise to celebrate my birthday. Of course, I charged the whole damn thing on my shiny new card. (Note to self: *not a good idea!*) It was a seven-day cruise departing from Miami. We sailed from one tropical paradise to the next, sightseeing, snorkeling, and day drinking at the beaches. We also reveled in our time at sea. Participating in passenger contests and pool games kept us entertained. We didn't want to go back to reality; the travel bug had definitely bitten me.

The following summer, on a whim, our next escapade took us to California. We barely had enough funds for the flight and not much cash when we got there. We hadn't made a plan as to where we'd stay when we arrived or how we would get around. Miraculously, we were conveniently seated next to a good-looking, friendly guy on the plane. He was single and just happened to live in Los Angeles. (Hmm … what a coincidence.)

During conversation we told him of our impulsive "adventure". Naive and desperate, we accepted his offer to stay at his place.

Shortly after arriving at his house, we realized that his plan was for all of us to share one bed! Eventually the awkward moment of going to bed was upon us. He quickly gave it a bold attempt, but we slept in our clothes and managed to avoid his hands all night. He was not exactly a "happy camper" when he dropped us off at the beach the next morning.

CHAPTER 2

Come Sail Away

It was late fall. Tina and I wanted to take a road trip before chilly winter weather arrived.

We had both been working a lot, and we were looking forward to the weekend getaway. The three-hour drive would take us to a big city complete with an amusement park. At some point during our trip, I needed to find a restroom. We came upon a truck stop, and pulled into the parking lot. I was about to pee my pants, so I jumped out and ran to the restaurant door without putting on my shoes. Opening the door, I noticed a sign that said "No Shirt, No Shoes, No Service." I barely stepped thru the door when the hostess, who didn't appear to be in a good mood, stopped me. "You are not allowed in here without shoes on!" she shouted at me. (She could have said it a little more nicely.) Okay, so now I had no choice but to go back to the car and put on my shoes. By this time, my bladder was ready to burst.

Returning to the restaurant, I finally made my way back to the ladies' room. What a relief! Then I felt the urge for a little fun. With Tina begging me not to, I swiftly took off my shirt and my bra. (Remember... "No Shirt, No Shoes ...") Then, exiting the bathroom topless, I calmly strolled through the restaurant, walked slowly past the hostess desk with a big toothy smile, and marched out the door. I couldn't help but notice that forks and spoons paused in midair as patrons' jaws dropped in disbelief. However, I have to admit, the minute I touched that door I ran my ass off! Tina had gone out before me and was starting the car as I jumped in. She stepped on the gas and we drove off as fast as we could! I still have to laugh when I think about the stunned look on the face of that hostess! We now refer to this café as the "breastaurant."

Of course, this was prior to the cell phone era. The outcome would definitely be different today. There would be video, and I would be in a lot of trouble!

The fun and games were a great distraction, but reality always eventually floats to the surface. The phrase "the only constant in life is change" was ringing true for me. At twenty-five years old, I was disillusioned, having learned the hard way that life isn't always the way you want it to be.

I knew that Tina and I could not continue to be roommates. Our relationship had become strained; there was an elephant in the room. Previously during a serious conversation, she had unexpectedly blurted out that she wanted to be more than friends. I am open minded and would never judge anyone on his or her sexuality, so in theory this shouldn't have been a problem, but in some weird way I felt betrayed, as if a sister had kept a big secret from me. I didn't have romantic feelings for her. Things became awkward, and our relationship quickly deteriorated.

It was heartbreaking, painful, and seemed like another divorce. Regrettably, we weren't able to mend our friendship. It is true that sometimes you have to let people go; not everyone is meant to stay.

At the beauty salon one morning, I was standing near the reception desk when Ali walked in the door. She was one of my boss's established hair clients, but she was scheduled with me for nail overlays that day. We exchanged greetings, and made our way through the salon to the nail area. As we settled into our chairs, Ali's wittiness already had me laughing. Seated at the small manicure table, conversation somehow led to our respective situations and became personal. She had just gone through a divorce and had a young daughter. I shared that I needed to move and was currently looking for an apartment.

We discovered a common bond—we were both going through a personal transition and concerned about finances. We talked about the possibility of becoming roommates. Ali had a newly built, three-bedroom home and was considering a housemate to help with expenses. Impulsively, we moved forward with a plan; I moved in three weeks later.

Ali was dazzling in so many ways. She couldn't enter a room without being noticed. People were instantly disarmed by her endearing and engaging manner. She was beautiful, kindhearted, and seldom missed an opportunity to insert a compliment into the conversation. Her festive sense of humor never failed to provide an entertaining perspective on whatever situation might arise!

Despite the stress of our respective circumstances, we tried to be positive and filled the house with laughter. After a particular evening out with friends, Ali was having trouble navigating the stairs to her bedroom. As she lay there on the landing, she remembered that it is not a good idea to skip dinner if you are going to indulge in cocktails! As I handed her small chunks of bread, we got the giggles because I had recently learned the same lesson. That night, our mantra became "just because you look like a lady, doesn't mean you have to act like one."

From day one, Ali and her daughter made me feel at home. We became family. (Sorry for not always being a good role model, kiddo, but you turned out just fine!)

I wasn't exactly rational on the day I bought the Camaro. Needing a dependable car, I was looking for something practical and inexpensive. Then, while walking the lot with the salesman, I saw it. I was just going to sit in that sports car for a minute, just for fun. Then something took over my brain.

Combining under budgeting and over spending is never a good idea. The happiness of driving that spicy-red Camaro faded as I struggled to make the car payments. Trying to salvage my credit rating, I called the loan company. "I am not able to pay the full amount that is due. Can we work something out?" I asked. I was too far behind, and they weren't in the mood to negotiate. A few days later, they responded with an official letter. My car was being repossessed. Someone would be coming to take it away.

Feeling like a failure, I spent most of that night in the garage sitting behind the wheel, sobbing like a little baby. This was becoming a pattern in my life—losing things. I had lost my mom, my marriage, my roommate, my apartment, and now my car.

Finally, after hours of sulking and feeling sorry for myself, exhausted and mentally numb, I tiptoed inside and crawled into bed.

At this point in life, I was thinking about starting a new career. Growing restless, I resolved to get a degree in fashion merchandising. That meant going back to school. I was taking classes in the morning, working at the salon in the afternoon, and waiting tables at night. It was a crazy schedule, but I was determined!

However, it wasn't all work and no play; I did manage to squeeze in a little social time! One Friday evening after work, some friends and I decided to meet at the Safari Club for drinks. We were on the dance floor being silly when I saw a good-looking guy with great hair sitting at the bar; he was wearing a suit jacket and tie. I noticed that he looked rather introspective and appeared to be by himself.

We made eye contact and, of course, I flashed my best flirtatious smile. As the song ended, my friends and I made our way back to the table. We were busy chatting. At some point, I felt a presence behind me and I looked up to see "Mr. Great Hair" behind me. Alan's clever pick up line: "I just have to dance with a girl who is brave enough to wear silver cowboy boots. Would you like to dance?" Of course I said yes! Later, as we were all getting ready to leave, he asked for my number. We made our way outside to wait for the valet. I was quite impressed when the valet pulled up in Alan's car. It was a brand-new burgundy Porsche 911. (I was, at that point, "rockin" an older model Datsun.)

A few months and many laughs later, one of us fell in love (that would be me). In fairness to me, our first date was on Valentine's Day. Alan was a successful marketing executive but decided to leave the corporate world to pursue a career in stand-up comedy. I had visions of a committed relationship, but his dreams of being a comedian didn't include me. Our lives were headed in different directions. He eventually moved to California.

Weary and disheartened, I was growing tired of the whole dating game. It takes a lot of energy both physically and mentally. I was also gaining weight, and that was really bringing me down. For some insane reason, I started taking laxatives and diuretics, thinking it would help me take off the pounds. When that didn't do the trick, I started making myself throw up after eating. I would frequently swallow a dose of ipecac after meals. Also during this phase, I decided that having a dark tan was a priority. I basked in the sun without sun block every chance I got, plus I used a tanning bed almost daily.

I ignored the fact that diuretics and UV rays are not a good mix. Water blisters would pop up on my legs, arms, and hands. They weren't painful, but would drain and disappear. At the same time, I was getting so dark that I did not realize I was developing freckles all over my arms and legs. As you might imagine, all this was taking a toll on my health.

My sister, Lynn, is a nurse. Unsurprisingly, it is her nature to be nurturing. Just six years older than I, she became my refuge when our mom died. As close as we are, I was embarrassed and hesitated to tell her what I was doing. I knew I should stop. My body had become dependent on the medications; when I didn't take them, my body overreacted and retained fluid. It was a catch twenty-two. Miserable, I eventually confided in Lynn. She insisted I meet with a friend of hers who was a doctor. He convinced me that I was on a dangerous path and was damaging my body. I trusted him and believed he could help me find the strength I needed. It didn't happen overnight, but with the doctor's guidance and my sister's support, I was able to stop taking the diuretics and quit purging. It was a slow dawning of understanding; over time I could look at myself in the mirror and see past the extra pounds. The illogical part was that, to anyone else, the weight was minimal.

Life is full of retrospection. We all have those voices in our heads that make us self-critical and insecure. Thankfully, I've had no desire to revisit those self-destructive habits. I can now appreciate and accept my body. I try to be kind to it.

My schedule was hectic and the days were long. Late one afternoon, I drove home from class, went upstairs, and melted on the floor next to my bed. Emotionally and spiritually spent, I wondered why my life was such a mess. I did not see a way out of debt, and I was exhausted from trying to balance school and work. My fashion class was taking a trip to New York City. The agenda included an insider's view of the garment district, and the expedition was a fundamental part of our curriculum. The cost was five hundred dollars, and I did not have it. I would be the only one in our class not going. I felt like a failure.

Ali overheard me in my room bawling uncontrollably and came rushing in to see what was wrong. Curled up in a fetal ball on the floor, I was crying so hard my body was convulsing. She knelt down beside me and held me in her arms until I ran out of tears.

The next morning I awoke to find an envelope on my dresser with $500 inside; there was a note from Ali saying it was a gift. I didn't want to accept it, but I did.

After graduating, the best job I could find was working in a retail store for minimum wage. Seriously? I was definitely questioning my decision to pursue a career in fashion merchandising.

It was time to make a drastic change. I couldn't continue on this path. Mulling over my options, I remembered the Caribbean cruise Tina and I had taken. I kept thinking how much fun it would be to work on a cruise ship. Plus, it would be expense free, and I'd be able to save money. Most ships have salons onboard. I decided to apply for a hairstylist position. Why not? Once I updated my resume, I sent copies to the popular cruise lines. After I made numerous (way too many) calls to the office of the crewing manager of a major cruise line, his assistant informed me, "Mr. Fisher has asked me to tell you that we are not hiring any hairstylists now or in the near future." I thought, *Great, I've pissed him off to the point that he won't even take my calls!*

Then, astonishingly, a couple weeks later, I got a call. "Hello, this is Mr. Fisher with [he mentioned the cruise line], and I have a job for you on one of our new vessels if you can be here on Saturday." (I found out later that someone had quit, and they were in a bind.) Of course, I jumped at the chance and accepted the position. Saturday was only three days away, but I didn't care I was going to do whatever it took to make this happen. I knew I had to take this chance if I wanted my life to change.

I quit both of my jobs, packed my clothes, and made arrangements with my sister to pick up the stuff I couldn't take with me. The cruise line had made arrangements for me to fly to Miami, Florida and join the ship there. I was in the middle of a whirlwind! The hardest part was saying good-bye to my family and friends.

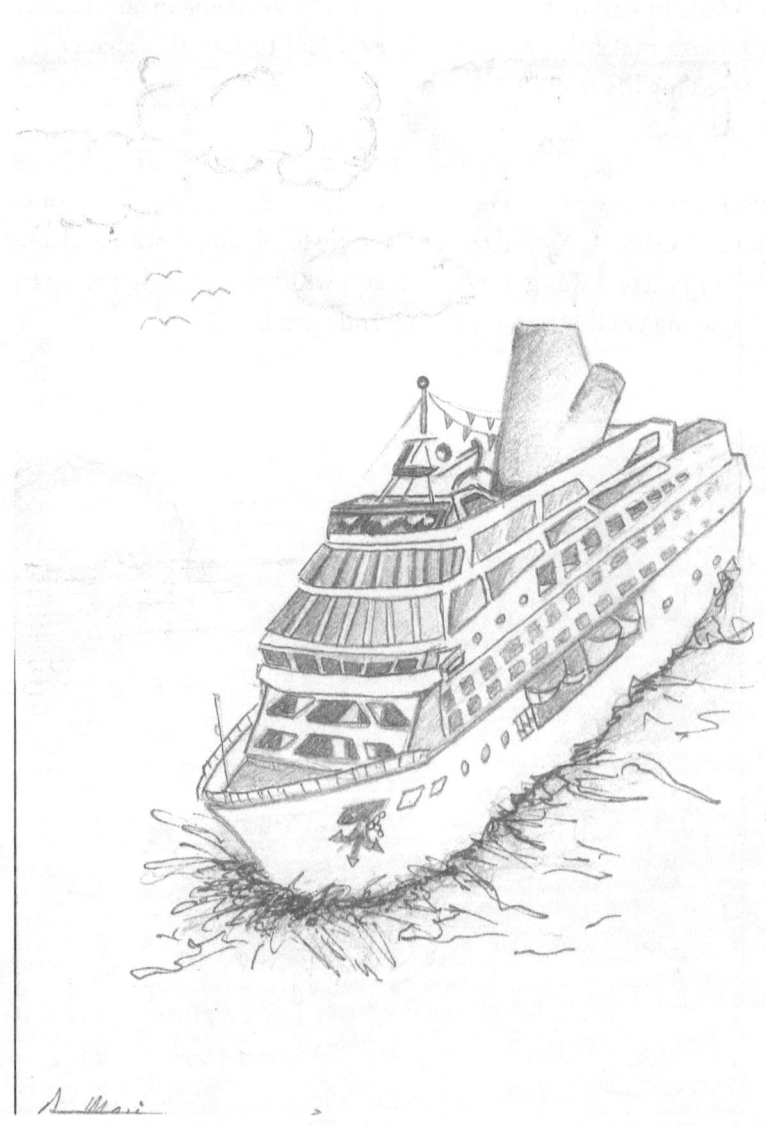

CHAPTER 3

Did I Sign Up for This?

The plane ride to Miami seemed endless. A mixture of apprehension and exhilaration stirred in my mind. When the pilot finally touched down at the airport, I was both jittery and anxious to get off the plane. Following the signs, I promptly made my way to the baggage claim area to collect my luggage. Arrangements had been made for someone to meet me and transport me to the cruise terminal. Scanning the sea of people, I spotted a man (looking bored) holding a sign with my name on it. As I approached him and introduced myself, he simply nodded and grabbed my bags. We made our way outside to find his car. As we passed through the automatic door, leaving the air-conditioning behind, the tropical humidity felt like I had stepped into a sauna. The heat slapped my face as I inhaled the moisture in the air. With my bags stowed in the trunk, Mr. Driver started the car and mumbled something about it being a short distance.

At last we were approaching the port of Miami, and I spotted the vessel tethered at the dock. She looked huge—she was gigantic! Besieged with anxiety and conflicting emotions, I started to feel sick to my stomach. Immediately after I'd gone through the security check-in process, an official-looking gentleman in a white uniform appeared and escorted me to the crew gangway. As I took that first step onto the metal walkway, my thought was, *Am I really doing this?* The doorway spilled into a wide corridor with a web of nondescript passages. I couldn't believe I was really there. I had actually got a job working on a cruise ship! I remember thinking, *Hope this Nebraska girl doesn't get seasick!*

The officer stationed at the gangway spoke into his radio, requesting a steward. My legs felt shaky as I was guided to the crew purser's office for processing. She smiled with a friendly hello and introduced herself as Lena. During our conversation, I learned that she was from Texas and this was her first ship as well. Lena was spirited and funny. I already knew we would be friends. After I completed the paperwork and acquired my crew badge, the cabin steward reappeared to take me to my cabin. The hallways were very narrow, and it was like walking thru a maze. I was wondering if I'd be able to find my way out of there. The steward eventually set my luggage down outside a door. Before disappearing, he kindly uttered "Good luck" with a foreign accent that I didn't recognize.

Opening the door, I peered into the smallest room I had ever seen. There were two cot-sized bunk beds, a built-in desk, a mini bathroom, and two tiny closets. There was just enough space for one person to walk between the bed and the closet. My roommate was stretched out on the bottom bunk. *Guess that means I am on the top one*, I thought. When I said hello, she glanced at my two overstuffed suitcases. "I don't know where you think you are going to put all of that," she said somewhat sarcastically. "I guess I over packed," I replied nervously. "I wasn't sure what I would need." Turned out she was right—I had to send most of it back home.

The first chance I had to call home was a few days later when the ship docked in St. Thomas. Finding the call center (typically located near the pier), I managed to place a brief call to my sister, Faye. "I hate it!" I complained. "I feel like I have joined the navy. The workdays are long, and there are so many rules." She empathetically replied, "Hang in there and give it some time." What other choice did I have? I had signed a six-month contract.

My first itinerary, or "run" as they say in the cruise ship industry, was the eastern Caribbean, including St. Thomas, St. Maarten, and San Juan. St. Thomas is known for great shopping; St. Maarten is famous for it's unconventional beaches. San Juan was typically an overnight port of call. Usually a group of crewmembers would meet somewhere for dinner and then find their way to one of the resort clubs for a night of dancing. It was during one of these excursions that I met Luca. He was a cadet officer onboard. He was tall, dark, and Italian! His English was excellent and his accent enticing. We danced our feet off and had a fun evening.

There is a distinction between ranks onboard the ship. There are officers, staff, and crew. Accommodations, privileges, and perks vary greatly depending upon a person's position. Officers have the fewest restrictions and the most perks. Staff members have restrictions but are allowed in passenger lounges and eateries. Crewmembers are not allowed in passenger areas when not on duty.

Since Luca was an officer and I was a staff member, we were both allowed to spend time eating, drinking, and socializing above crew deck. We enjoyed spending time together, and it didn't take long for us to become a couple.

Having finally adjusted to life onboard, I was enjoying my job and truly happy to be there. There were only four of us working in the salon, and we were close comrades. I became especially close to Stacey. She was also on her first contract and had only been onboard a few weeks. While the salon was open, we worked long hours, especially on formal nights. But when the salon was closed, we found the fun! On the nights we didn't feel like dressing for passenger areas, we stayed below on the crew deck. The crew areas are like another city beneath the passenger decks. The narrow passages are bland and bare, the cabins are small, and it's not unusual to see a crowd gathered for an impromptu party in a hallway. We spent a few nights perfecting our game of "quarters" in the crew bar, which was always a popular spot to hang out and de-stress.

Lena was not only the crew purser; she also worked at the shore excursion desk, which happened to come with some nice perks. She got to "try out" some excursions cost free. The local tour companies offered these opportunities in hopes that we would recommend their tours to the cruise passengers.

At sea one day Lena called me and asked, "I have tickets for four to take the helicopter island tour tomorrow. Want to go?" "Of course!" I exclaimed. "Sounds fun!" The next morning, we met our boyfriends at the gangway. Lena had arranged for a driver to take us to the local helicopter tour company.

The helicopter was waiting when we arrived, and we quickly climbed inside; we were all excited about this adventure! The pilot would actually leave us on the uninhabited island. We would be the only humans on the island until he returned for us three hours later!

From above, the island was breathtakingly beautiful and the surrounding ocean a transparent crystal blue. First we spent our time exploring the island; it was a strange feeling knowing we were stranded and totally dependent upon the helicopter coming back for us. Finished with that venture, we all laid our towels down on the beach and quickly devoured the picnic lunch we had brought with us.

After lunch, we had about half an hour before the pilot was supposed to return. What to do … what to do? Okay—we could not leave there without a little beach sexy time! Luca and I discovered the perfect place as we noticed Lena and her boyfriend disappearing down the sandy shore. We weren't in any hurry to hear those helicopter blades approaching!

Exploring new places was exciting for me. I was like a kid in a candy store. Passengers from all walks of life came and went, and conversations were multifarious. I was enjoying the lifestyle. I was content. Then unexpectedly, things changed.

That morning a few months into my contract, the salon manager asked the staff to arrive at the salon thirty minutes early. She had called a meeting to give us the news: "The salon contract has been assigned to an English company. Within a few weeks, we will no longer have our positions on board." Not wanting to leave, I felt crushed. We all did. The next day, we were informed that we would be dispersed to various ships to finish our contracts. The four of us were frustrated and very sad to be going our separate ways. Saying good-bye to everyone was tough, especially with Luca. I had just adjusted to ship life and now I was facing another new beginning. It was like moving to a new city, changing jobs, and making all new friends at the same time.

My transfer took me to a ship based in the port of Los Angeles; our itinerary included ports of call in Mexico. This ship was a few years older and quite a bit smaller. It didn't take long for me to realize that the salon manager wasn't thrilled to be inheriting me. Not one to hold back, she made it clear she had planned to hire someone else. She was frosty, and I was miserable. One afternoon, as I was grabbing a quick lunch (sitting alone in the crew mess), I looked across the room and recognized one of the entertainers onboard. Vic was a singer and had spent some time on my previous ship. It was comforting to see a familiar face. He joined me for lunch and—for that day—I felt a little less lonely. Settling into my new floating home was taking longer than I had expected.

Living at sea forces you to find creative ways to entertain yourself. On April Fools Day, I thought it would be fun to surprise Vic with a prank. Having seen his show a few times, I knew there was a point during a certain song when he would take off his leather jacket. My cohorts and I arrived at the lounge an hour early that night. We approached several female guests and asked if they would be willing to participate in our prank. Those willing to join in were asked to go to their staterooms, bring back a pair of their underwear, and wait for their cue.

As Vic was performing the song and started to make his sexy, trademark move of removing his jacket, a crowd of women rushed toward him and threw their panties onstage. He was so stunned that it took a few minutes for him to recover enough to continue with his set. Mission accomplished!

Patti worked in the spa as a massage therapist. She was energetic, quick to laugh, and not afraid to break the rules. One night we decided it would be fun to stay overnight in Puerto Vallarta and catch up with the ship the next day. We knew that flights between the ports would be available. Missing the ship was a big no-no and, almost without fail, resulted in being fired. Crew and staff were always required to be onboard one hour prior to the ship's departure.

Neither one of us had to work the next day, we felt sure our absence would not be discovered. We had an awesome night in Puerto Vallarta. We stayed in a hotel and, as planned, caught the plane the next day. The problem was that traffic in Mexico is unpredictable, and we had not allowed enough time for the drive from the airport. We arrived at the dock just in time to see the crew gangway pulled inside the ship. The passenger gangway was already gone, and the door was closed. Our only choice was to throw our bags onboard and jump the few feet from the dock into the ship. Luckily the ship had not yet pulled away and there were a couple crewmembers willing to help us onboard. I was never so glad to see my cabin!

With our contracts soon coming to an end, Patti and I discussed getting an apartment together in Los Angeles. Her brother and his wife had a house there and would let us stay with them while we look for a place. Not wanting to go back to Nebraska, I decided it sounded like a good plan.

Our last day onboard arrived, and we said our good-byes. You get close with people very quickly when working on ships because time seems to be condensed. It is comparable to living in a small town. The tough part is that people come and go constantly. That morning, with my future uncertain, I walked down the gangway feeling uneasy and sad. I did not look back at the ship. Patti's brother met us outside the port building and drove us to his house. I felt uncomfortable and wondered if I was really welcome.

First things first: buy a car and get a job. Patti and I were lucky enough to find jobs right away. A bus tour company was hiring tour operators to host groups to Lake Tahoe. Now, sometimes things sound a little better than they are. The reality was that we rode on buses filled with demanding senior citizens for hours at a time. The coach tour provided round trips from Los Angeles to Lake Tahoe. We had three days in Tahoe with casino tours and various activities. It was our job to entertain the guests as well as make sure that everything went according to schedule. If I never play another game of bingo, that will be fine with me!

Living with Patti at her brother's house became increasingly awkward. I didn't feel comfortable there, and I told her I wanted to move out. On one of my trips to Tahoe, I met a guide named Tasha. When she heard that I was looking for an apartment, she said she could use a roommate to share expenses.

It seemed there was more to her story, but I couldn't quite figure it out. With tension growing between Patti and me, moving sounded better and better. I packed everything I had into my frail, ancient car and made the drive to Tasha's house. It took longer than anticipated. I didn't have a GPS, and the directions she had given me were complicated. Tasha came flying out the door when I finally pulled into the short driveway. She was happy to see me, and I felt relieved. As she showed me around the small apartment, I was surprised to learn that my bed would be the sofa in the living room—and not even a pullout sofa!

Two weeks passed, and since we both worked long hours, we didn't see much of each other. Then one night I came home and quickly realized that Tasha had a guest in her bedroom. I changed into my pajamas and quietly crawled onto my "bed." Just as I was starting to doze off, suddenly Tasha was leaning over me as she whispered, "My friend asked if you would join us." I politely declined. The next day Tasha told me about her second job—she was a professional call girl and was hoping I'd be interested in earning some extra cash. As soon as she left for work, I grabbed my things, threw them in the car, and got the hell out of there!

Exasperated, I resorted to calling my cousin, who lived in a suburb of Los Angeles. Without pause, she invited me to stay with her until I could formulate a plan. I really wanted to continue working on ships. The travel bug had bitten me, and I actually missed the lifestyle. With nothing to lose, I applied to the company that had purchased the salon concession. Despite the fact that most of their employees were European, I was offered a contract. I felt as if I'd won the lottery! I was excited to be working for this well-known cruise line. This contract was onboard a ship that visited diverse ports of call in South America and included passing through the Panama Canal. The fifty-mile canal connects the Atlantic (Caribbean Sea) to the Pacific Ocean. Ships pass through a sequence of locks and passages; transit time can take eight to ten hours. It was fascinating to observe.

Salon crewmembers had the rank of staff, which meant that we were allowed to drink and socialize in the nightclub, but dancing was strictly forbidden. Dance floor space was reserved for passengers and officers. Throwing caution to the wind after a few cocktails, I was getting into the music and happily bounced onto the dance floor. Demonstrating my best moves, I felt liberated! That was until I looked over my shoulder to see the captain glaring at me. Melting into the crowd, I vanished as fast as I could. Early the next morning, I was summoned to the staff captain's office and informed that my consequence would be the suspension of my lounge privileges.

My next contract sent me to Alaska. The ship was smaller and significantly older than any vessel I had worked on. That fact became obvious as I walked through the crew halls and arrived at my shabby cabin. I wasn't thrilled to see that my cabin mate and I would be sharing a common bathroom with the cabin next door. That was definitely tricky when everyone needed to get ready for work.

The salon, like our cabin, was quite cozy. There was barely enough space for three of us. The other hairstylist was a fun-loving French Canadian who spoke four languages. Our British salon manager was hilarious. His sarcastic sense of humor entertained the passengers and ensured that the workday was never boring!

With each new contract, it became a little easier to acclimate. I acquired some degree of comfort in knowing what to expect of ship life, even though each ship was comparable to an unknown city with a new set of friends. Those first few days aboard were daunting and exhilarating at the same time. Curiously, instead of dreading change, I was motivated by it.

The beauty of Alaska is spectacular and awe inspiring. The massive glaciers are fascinating from afar and even more mesmerizing up close. There are helicopter tours that drop visitors off at the top base where tour guides emerge from a warm tent to take them on an expedition across the ice mass. During one of these ventures, as our group was returning to base camp, the fog rapidly thickened to the point of near zero visibility. It was too risky for the helicopters to come back for us. It was going to be a while. The temperature was dropping, and we were all freezing. Fortunately the guides' tent was equipped with a small heater, so they invited us to take turns warming up in the humble abode. At one point, the fog thinned slightly, but it was expected to increase in density. The pilots made the decision to make the attempt before conditions got worse. It was like a scene out of MASH. We heard the rumble of engines and whirl of the blades as four helicopters appeared through the fog. The plan was to take us to the nearest clearing below, as it was impossible to return to the airport. There would be a bus arriving to transport us from that location back to the ship. Thankfully the captain of our ship had been advised of the situation and had delayed departure. Who knew our excursion would leave us stranded on a glacier for three hours? Was this Gilligan's Glacier?

The end of that contract coincided with the ship going into dry dock. During dry dock the ship is floated into a basin of water, then the water is drained so that the vessel rests on a dry platform. This allows for maintenance and repairs of the ship. It was such a strange sight to see the ship (my home) out of the water. Walking off the ship and down the pier that day was the end of a chapter, and the good-byes were getting harder. During my contract breaks, I would usually go visit family in the Midwest. Typically I would work for six months and have a two-month break between contracts. Usually at the end of a break I was looking forward to going back. This time felt different. Maybe I needed a change of course.

During that break, I sent resumes to other cruise companies. When the executive with a Hawaii bases cruise line called, I was thrilled. Under the impression I had procured an onboard position,

I impulsively moved to Maui. Taking only what I could carry on the plane, I was excited and eager to see Hawaii. Unfortunately upon my arrival in Lahaina, it was abruptly apparent that the guy who hired me had been tricky and less than truthful. I was not being transported to the ship terminal. I would not being working onboard as promised. The position had somehow morphed into working at their resort salons on land.

I didn't know where I would sleep that night. I had to find a place to stay until I could sort out the situation. After a couple days at a hotel (and a fiery conversation with my new boss), I decided to stay and accept the position. Searching for an apartment, I stumbled upon an advertisement for a housemate. The rent would be $500 per month. I thought that was quite reasonable for Maui. I quickly learned why—I would be sharing the three- bedroom, one-bath home with another female and four guys!

Needing a place right away, I couldn't be too picky, so I hastily became the sixth tenant. My housemates were a group of peculiar individuals, each quirky in their own way. I did get the luxury of having my own bedroom, but my furniture consisted of a mattress on the floor and a wooden chair. One night I awoke to a strange sensation; I felt something crawling on me … lots of something crawling on me. I jumped up and hit the light switch. To my horror, I saw an army of ants—monstrously large red ants—all over my bed! Since I was screaming and thrashing about, a couple of the guys come running in to see what was wrong. They remained very calm and informed me that I was not allowed to kill the ants. The yogi of the group appeared with a vacuum and proceeded to relocate them outside. I was having second thoughts about my housing situation.

I bought myself a tatty old Ford for $500. Since I would be alternating between two resort salons, I needed transportation. The car had problems to say the least. But, thankfully, I didn't have to drive a long distance to work.

I definitely wasn't prepared for how expensive it was to live in Hawaii. It didn't take long to realize that my salary wasn't going to be enough to support myself. I needed a second income. The popular piano bar and restaurant down the street was hiring cocktail waitresses. I applied and luckily got the job. It was so close I could walk to work!

However, after months of working two jobs and barely making ends meet, I could no longer find a place for the word "fun" in my vocabulary. I was starting to hate "land life" and I started to rethink my decision to move to Hawaii. I had made friends and met some great people, but I was getting bored, and island fever was starting to consume me. After a lot of soul searching, I came to the conclusion that staying there wasn't going to work for me. Making the decision to leave was the easy part, but again, I had no plan.

There was one last thing I wanted to do before I left. I had to see the Haleakala volcano! Unsurprisingly, my old ford turned out to be sicker than I thought. She had a habit of leaking water from the radiator and overheating. This can be a major problem when you are forging up a constant incline to the top of a mountain. In preparation, I had brought a few jugs of water with me. Every so often, I had to stop the car, open the hood, and replenish the fluid in the radiator. Pure determination got me to the top, and when I finally saw it, emotion overcame me. It was an incredible sight, so deep and vast with rich shades of orange and brown soil. The energy felt sacred and majestic. That was one of the last ventures for my little heap of metal. But on a happy note, I was able to sell it for the same price I had paid for it!

I slept during most of that long flight back to the Midwest. When I awoke, my thoughts were focused on *"What am I going to do now?" and "I can't keep coming back to my sister".* One of the first to disembark, I was excited to see family. Spending time with them was restoring.

Not sure what direction my life was headed, I took a part-time job as a server at the local country club. I was making good money and it was something to do. However, it didn't take long for discontentment to sneak up on me. The job became boring and I was getting fidgety. Maybe I wasn't ready to clip my wings.

CHAPTER 4

The Wonder of Waves

While researching cruise lines, I discovered a brand new luxury cruise line. They were hiring crewmembers for their first vessel. The ships were significantly smaller with a capacity of only one hundred passengers. It sounded intriguing, and I couldn't have placed that resume in the mail any faster. A week had passed, that morning I came home after going for a run and checked the voicemail. I had a message. The director had received my resume and wanted to speak with me. With shaky fingers, I dialed the number. "The person we previously hired for the position is unable to fulfill the commitment. How soon could you join the ship in Italy?" Before the conversation was over, I had the job and a flight reservation. I was beyond ecstatic! I had a plan, a purpose. I couldn't believe I was going to Europe! Arriving a few days later, I met up with the rest of the crew at a hotel near the shipyard in Italy. Knowing that the rest of the crew had arrived a week or two before me was a little intimidating. Everyone knew each other and I was "late to the party". To make matters worse, the airline had lost my luggage. It was days before it caught up with me! The crewing manager kindly arranged for me to choose some clothes from the ship's boutique. They weren't quite my style, but wearing them was definitely better than being stuck in my travel clothes for the rest of the week!

The pristine vessel was docked in the harbor ready for her maiden voyage. By the time the mooring lines were untied and we were pulling away from the dock, I already felt like part of the team. Everyone was excited to be embarking on this new adventure.

My position was salon and boutique manager; I divided my time between the two. Being the only hairstylist onboard, I had a captive clientele! The boutique was located on the main deck in a high-traffic area near the passenger services desk. Throughout the cruise most everyone passing by would stop in to say hello and check out the merchandise. Except for the constant refolding of clothing, I enjoyed working there, using those fashion merchandising skills after all!

Onboard accommodations required the hairdresser to share a cabin with two cabin mates, both stewardesses. Their bunk beds were at one end of the room, and mine was a slightly larger bed at the other end. There wasn't much space between the foot of the bunk beds and the headboard of mine; a curtain between them provided some privacy. Sharing such limited space with cabin mates usually works out okay, you learn to adapt.

This stunning yacht-like vessel was three hundred feet in length. The overall capacity included one hundred passengers and seventy multi-national crewmembers. Her maiden voyage took us to extraordinary places. Many mornings I would wake up in yet a different part of the world. Due to her size, the small ship was able to call on unique places like quaint villages and tiny seaside towns, not accessible by bigger vessels.

When the ship was in port, the salon and boutique were closed. Being a runner, I found that my favorite way to discover a new port was to take off on a long run. Naively overlooking the fact that I was in a foreign country, I ran through cities in Yemen and Egypt wearing only running shorts and a tank top. I didn't consider that my clothing (or lack thereof) went against religious customs and I could be putting myself in danger. In retrospect, my behavior was disrespectful, and I certainly would do things differently today.

During that contract I met Paolo, a deck officer. What had started as playful flirtation soon evolved into an intimate relationship. Time is accelerated when living on ships, partially because everyone has a finite period of time onboard. Not only do you work together, you are living in the same "house." Ship life is a giant step away from the reality of life. It is life in a bubble. I wish I could say I didn't know he was married, but I did.

Some people who work onboard ships are there for the money; others are there for the adventure. I was there for both. I wanted to see the world. When I walked down that gangway onto the pier in a place I had never been before, I would feel a rush of excitement. My shipmates and I would sometimes take an organized shore excursion, but more often than not, we would explore on our own.

The ships croupier—casino dealer—was from Scotland and was always up for a good adventure. Upon our arrival in Beppu, Japan, we had a fun day planned. The city of Beppu is nestled between the mountains and the sea. It is famous for *onsens*—hot springs mud baths. We hired a taxi to take us to the resort. At first it was odd to see people naked and covered with mud, but we wanted the authentic experience and promptly followed suit. As we approached the muddy pit, we noticed a couple of the elderly ladies trying to get our attention. We eventually understood that they were telling us to cover our "lady parts" with our hands (mud bath etiquette 101).

It was easy to become an adrenaline junkie, every port offered new scenery, exploration, and adventure. Crewmembers have a way of finding places away from the typical tourist path.

A few months had passed when I heard the current chief purser would be transferring to another ship, which meant her position would be open. Contacting the corporate office, I requested to be considered as her replacement. When they responded that they would approve the promotion, I was beyond ecstatic and eager to prove myself. The chief purser was the officer to whom I reported. We had become friends, so when the task of training me fell upon her, she was graciously supportive.

The chief purser reported directly to the hotel manager and was responsible for the onboard safe and the handling of company monies. This included passenger statements and payments as well as crew payroll. In addition to manning the reception desk, it was my duty to clear the ship whenever we arrived in port. There were specific requirements in each port that had to be met before anyone was allowed to disembark. It was my job to prepare all necessary forms along with current passenger and crew manifests. As soon as we docked, immigration officials would come onboard, and I would provide any required documentation and passports. Most clearances went smoothly, but not every time. I remember the day we docked at the Russian port of Leningrad. I greeted the Immigration and Custom officials, as they filed onboard. Escorting them to the lounge where we would begin the clearance process, I invited them to take their seats at the table. The official in charge rudely barked, "We want to meet with the Chief Purser". The look on their faces when I informed them that I was the Chief Purser was bewilderment. Apparently they were not accustomed to working with female officers, and they were not happy about it. After I presented the required clearance forms and all documentation they requested, they stated that they would have one more requirement. In order to clear the vessel they would require "a gift" in cases of eggs.

If that's what it was going to take to give us passage, then eggs they shall have! They were a happier bunch when they walked back down that gangway. It was always a relief when we were granted entry and we could begin disembarkation!

When the small ship was sailing through areas of potential pirate threats, we took extra precautions and had to be aware of inherent danger. It made me feel uneasy; we kept a significant amount of cash in the office, and I was the one who held the combination to the safe.

With the rank of officer, being chief purser definitely had its perks, including a large cabin, a bar allowance, and few restrictions onboard. As long as my work was done, I was free to go ashore when the ship was in port. But I definitely earned my wages on turnaround day—disembarkation/embarkation. On those days, it was not unusual for me to work more than fifteen hours straight.

When I needed solitude, I loved to find a secluded spot outside on deck and just watch the hypnotic waves roll by. There was something therapeutic about looking out over the massive ocean and being surrounded by sea with no land in sight. It is true that the sea is good for the soul!

As I reflect back on my time aboard cruise ships, I still feel a sense of awe at the incredible places I was privileged to see. How many of us have hiked on a dirt trail among komodo dragons on Komodo Island? Explored the pyramids at Giza? Or stood amongst the pumice stones on the streets of Pompeii? Touring the atomic bomb museums in Hiroshima and Nagasaki made an imprint on my soul. The evidence of the resulting devastation was overpowering. The horrendous photos of injured people were unbearable.

When visiting other countries, I made an effort to explore the various cultures. Usually that meant sightseeing, browsing through shops, or dining at one of the offbeat restaurants. I enjoyed interacting with the local people; it was fascinating and educational.

In the port of Istanbul, Turkey, my curiosity led me to a Turkish bath house. I convinced another crewmember to go with me. The bathing rooms were housed in a large stone building. When we entered our designated room, we were surprised to see that it was not divided by gender. The grey walls were lined with cement benches. We squeezed into our seats wearing only our towels. When it came to my turn, I was summoned to the washing area at one end of the room. The attendant first washed and rinsed my hair. Then she proceeded to bathe every inch of my body. I thought it would be awkward, but it wasn't. The practice is so natural for them. The public *hammam*, which provides a spa-like experience, is still a major part of the culture.

When our ship was docked at Port Said, Egypt, our itinerary included an overnight stay. This was scheduled to accommodate passengers who wanted to travel to Giza and tour the pyramid complex. The trip took two to three hours by car each way.

Of course, we crewmembers took advantage of this too! Four of us crammed into the tiny taxi. We couldn't be that close and not go see the most mysterious ancient monuments in the world! The Great Pyramid was awe-inspiring; we reverently navigated the passages and explored the stone chambers.

Before heading back to our taxi, we ended our excursion with the compulsory camel photo, which, by the way, made me want a shower. He was sweaty and smelled bad. The drive to the pyramids had passed quickly because we were excited and full of chatter. However, the ride back to the ship was long and scary. The sun had set, and the desert road was in total blackness. Urging our driver, who barely spoke any English, to turn on the headlights, my friend pulled out her flashlight and pointed to the front of the car. He matter-of-factly said, "No work." "What?" we all asked in unison. Without a hint of concern, he accelerated and maintained high speeds on the barely visible road. White-knuckling anything we could hold onto, we were paralyzed in fear. Finally back at the ship, we wondered if he had purposely been having fun at our expense.

That road trip was scary, but I can't recall a more terrifying circumstance than being caught in a typhoon, as our ship headed for Japan. Since it was a repositioning cruise, we did not have passengers onboard. The howling wind was fierce and deafening. We were miles from any shore when the ship lost all power and the backup generators failed. The yacht-sized ship was bobbing aimlessly like a rubber duck in a bathtub. In the moonlight, the waves were black and massive. At some point, an enormous and powerful wall of water crashed over the bow, cracking the bridge window. The ship started rolling from side to side, each roll more terrifying than the one before. The lack of lighting made movement dangerous. Petrified crewmembers huddled together, praying we wouldn't capsize. Everything that wasn't bolted down was flying off shelves and desks, including television sets.

More than twenty-four hours after the storm had passed, a tow vessel was finally able to reach us and drag our disabled ship to shore. I may have kissed the ground that day!

Taking a turn to the fun side of things...Who doesn't love a good April fool's hoax? It was springtime and we were sailing the Caribbean. April fools day was approaching, and Rita was looking to prank her husband. I didn't have to be asked twice!

Jon and Rita were married; he was the cruise director, and she was the shore excursion manager. Each time we docked at a particular renowned Caribbean island, I met with two local officials to clear the ship, and Rita worked with them on shore with regard to excursion issues. We had developed a friendly rapport with them, so when we asked for a favor they were willing to help us out. The plan unfolded perfectly. I was to frantically convey to Jon that his wife had been arrested and was being detained on the island. I must have done a good job of it because, distressed and in shock, he couldn't get there fast enough. We jumped in a taxi. When we arrived at the detention center, an officer greeted us and agreed to let us talk with her. As we made our way down the old stone stairs to the cell area, Jon's face was turning white. The jail was very old; the cement walls were stark and the air chilling. Finally we stood before a cell. There was Rita sitting behind bars. Poor Jon—we may have taken this too far! Unable to continue the charade, Rita and I burst into laughter, divulging it was all a prank. Now, that was fun for us, but not necessarily for him. He vowed revenge, and he certainly got it a few days later!

To make sure all paperwork was in order for ship clearance, I would typically be in my office well ahead of our arrival in any port. Our ETA (expected time of arrival) on this particular morning was seven o'clock. Just before four in the morning, my phone began to ring. As I picked up, I heard Jon anxiously shouting, "We are arriving now, and the officials will be onboard any minute! Hurry! Hurry!" After leaping out of bed and haphazardly throwing on my uniform, I literally ran downstairs to the reception desk and sprinted toward my office. But I stopped suddenly when Jon and his recruited cohorts jumped up from behind the reception desk and, in unison, shouted "April Fools!"

CHAPTER 5

Seventy Countries

My final contract took me to South America. After five years of travel at sea, I began to feel that the lifestyle was losing its appeal. Instead of being excited about a new contract, I was dreading it.

The ship was calling on ports in Chile as the last day of my commitment approached. I disembarked in Puerto Montt. It was a three-hour drive to the airport in Punta Arenas across dirt roads with hardly any traffic. The driver didn't speak a word of English. I started to consider my vulnerability and had to force myself to think about something else. Sometime during that lengthy journey, I made the decision that I didn't want to work on ships anymore. I was so done with starting over—tired of new beginnings, confined spaces, and draining good-byes. The onset of every contract was like moving to a new city and starting a new job every six months; it took a lot of energy. My travels had taken me to more than seventy countries, including countless ports, cities, and villages. It had been a great way to see the world, but I was tired of living out of a suitcase. Every worldly possession I owned fit in a three by six foot closet.

Having heard that corporate headquarters in Florida was planning to hire an assistant to the vice president in marine operations; I didn't hesitate to contact the office to let them know I was interested in the position. Later that week, I was back on a plane, this time on my way to meet with the hiring executive. I'm sure that having worked onboard gave me the advantage over other applicants, but the interview went well, and I was thrilled to land (pun intended) the job.

I was beyond excited about moving to Florida! A friend I had worked with onboard ships was living in an apartment near Fort Lauderdale Beach. She graciously offered to let me stay with her while I looked for my own place. Luckily it didn't take long for me to find an apartment. It was more expensive than I had hoped, but it was perfect—and furnished!

At first, performing my administrative duties and learning about marine operations was stimulating. But the transition to "land life" was more complex than I had anticipated. Sitting behind a desk all day quickly lost its luster. I missed the thrill of waking up in a foreign country. I missed the adventure. Also, I was having a hard time making my rent payment. I'd always been a slow learner when it came to budgeting. I never had to worry about room and board expenses when I lived on ships!

Paolo had also left ship life and was living with his wife in a house near my apartment. We continued to see each other occasionally. On a rainy day that summer, the gloomy skies matched my mood. Our afternoon rendezvous left me feeling empty and immoral. We said good-bye as I closed the door behind him. The onus hit me like a brick wall: I couldn't do this anymore. Suddenly nauseous, I sprinted through my apartment to the bathroom. Barely making it to the toilet, I threw up. Maybe it was a symbolic purging of all the emotion. I felt tremendous guilt knowing he had a wife. It never feels good to be second choice, and I could only blame myself for being in that situation. Curled up on that bathroom floor, I wondered if I would ever be "good enough" to be someone's first choice.

Was this karma for the pain I had caused those left in my wake? I hadn't considered the consequences of my selfishness. There was a hole in my life, and I felt completely alone. It was my darkest moment, I considered going to the beach, walking into the ocean, and not stopping. I dropped on my knees and pleaded with God to bring some joy to my life. I wanted someone special to share my life with.

Looking back on those years, I realize that true contentment was elusive. I wasn't afraid to pick up and move to unknown places. I was tough on the outside, but on the inside I was looking for acceptance and validation. I now regret measuring my worth by others' perception of me. I've also learned that things don't always come to be when we think they should. Sometimes things feel frozen because they are meant to be.

A powerful mantra to keep in mind:
You do enough. You have enough. You are enough.

I vividly remembered my first encounter with a psychic, which had taken place so many years ago. As I had walked slowly into the room, my heart had been beating wildly. Did I really want to know my future? My past had been painful in many ways, and I imagined there would be painful times embedded in the fabric of my life to come.

Recently divorced and unsure of my future, I'd been hoping for something to look forward to. I wasn't sure what to expect, so when she greeted me at the door, I was relieved to see a welcoming, silver-haired woman. As we sat across from each other at the small round table, she stunned me with the things she knew. Years later, after I had forgotten much of the reading, something stuck in my mind. I would marry again. She told me we would meet "in passing." She said, "He will be wearing a dark suit. His hair is dark and there is something about his voice … He has a deep voice." That had been ten years ago.

Now in my thirties, I was starting to crave some stability in my life. One of my responsibilities as the marine operations assistant was to acquire quotes for fuel prices from brokers for bunkering (fueling) the vessels. Prior to the ship's arrival in a port where they would require fuel, I would contact fuel broker companies for price quotes, usually by calling them on the phone. One broker was particularly charming and quick-witted. We progressed to some flirting during our conversations. I loved his voice and his sense of humor. This continued for a few months. Then, one morning, he was scheduled to visit our office for a meeting with my boss. When the receptionist rang to say he had arrived, I happily sprinted downstairs to greet him and escort him to the marine department. He was very attractive; his navy suit fit perfectly. He had dark hair and exuded confidence. "He is quite tasty," I whispered to my coworker.

The psychic's words from so long ago rushed into my thoughts, and I wondered if I had just met "him." A few days later we met for a business dinner. That dinner lasted five hours! Due to our professional relationship, we were a bit cautious about jumping into a personal relationship, but not for long! Marco was well traveled, and we had a wow-like connection. On the evenings we weren't together, we spent hours talking on the phone.

Looking to advance my career and wanting more of a challenge, I had been looking into opportunities with other companies. Eventually a renowned ship management company offered me the crew operator position. I was ecstatic! My new responsibilities varied from maintaining crewmember contract schedules to procuring visas. The job required some travel. Diversity in the workday made the job stimulating, and I was much more content.

Marco and I were married within the year. Our son, James, was born less than a month after our first anniversary, and fourteen months later our daughter, Leah, joined the family. The following year was a blur, and sleep became a much-sought-after commodity! For a short time, my nieces took turns living with us to nanny while I went back to work, but they were young and had to get back to their lives.

After evaluating everything and assessing our childcare options, we made the decision that I would put my career on hold to stay home and care for our children.

A few months after Leah was born, my sister Faye and her husband had planned to come visit and spend time with our little ones. They insisted that Marco and I plan a getaway to enjoy some leisure time and regenerate. We happily accepted their offer! Marco and I had met, married, and had two children all within three years. We needed some downtime!

Wanting adventure and looking for somewhere fun to go, I wondered what it would be like to visit a nudist resort. On a whim, I booked the reservation. (I didn't divulge that detail of our destination to my sister.)

Marco found it hilarious that I was packing so much stuff to go to a nudist resort. After a two-hour drive, we arrived at our destination. It was larger than we expected. In addition to the hotel, there were apartments and homes for full-time residents. As we drove through the unclothed community, I noticed bodies of all ages, shapes, and sizes. I was impressed that they seemed so comfortable with themselves. We saw an elderly woman tending to her garden wearing nothing but shoes; that could be a tad awkward when the grandkids come to visit! Then a middle-aged man in his birthday suit zipped past us driving a golf-cart.

We parked at the reception office, checked in, and found our way to our room. As we set down our things, it hit me! Turning to Marco

I shrieked, "Oh, God, we have to take our clothes off to leave this room!" Apprehension mixed with fear suddenly filled the air.

After finally summoning the courage to disrobe, we left the security of our hotel room, grabbing our towels as we stepped out the door. The resort information had stated that everyone is required to place a towel on the chair before taking a seat. This was proper etiquette for good hygiene. I kept fighting the urge to wrap that towel around my "lady business"! With map in hand, we walked down the street and over to the pool area. A naked man waved as he rode by on his bicycle (now there is a visual for you!).

We opened the door to walk inside the sunny pool bar and were relieved to see it wasn't crowded. Hurriedly finding a table near the wall, we placed the required towels on the seats and planted our butts on the chairs. The bartender was polite and fixed his gaze on our faces as he asked, "What would you like to drink?" I was thinking I needed a triple something, but heard myself say, "Gin and tonic, please." Marco ordered some "foo-foo" frozen drink (I always tease him when he does that). Feeling awkward, we focused on playing a game of backgammon. We enjoyed a relaxing afternoon. By dinnertime we were feeling somewhat comfortable in our new environment. That is, until we arrived at the restaurant and discovered it was a buffet. Check that one off the bucket list!

The years came and went. Life got busy. We moved our little family to a small seaside town in Florida. I never resumed that career in the marine industry; the corporate world no longer enticed me. Actively involved with volunteer organizations, I felt blessed to be a full-time mom. Life felt perfect.

After experiencing a Reiki treatment at a day spa, I became interested in holistic healing. The potential of alternative therapies was fascinating. Based on the concept that there are energy centers called chakras associated with the physical body, Usui Reiki is an ancient Japanese technique that promotes healing. During the relaxing treatment, vital energy is channeled to restore balance when energy has been disrupted or blocked by injury or disease. Curiously intrigued, I signed up for Reiki courses, eventually obtaining my Reiki Master certification.

The process further opened my mind to the connection of mind, body, and spirit. Striving for optimal health, the holistic approach takes the whole person into account rather than focusing on a particular symptom or part of the body.

In May of 2011, James and Leah were in their last years of high school and preparing to leave for college. Marco and I were starting to wonder what the next chapter of our lives would bring.

And then...I was diagnosed with breast cancer.

PART TWO

My Personal Journal

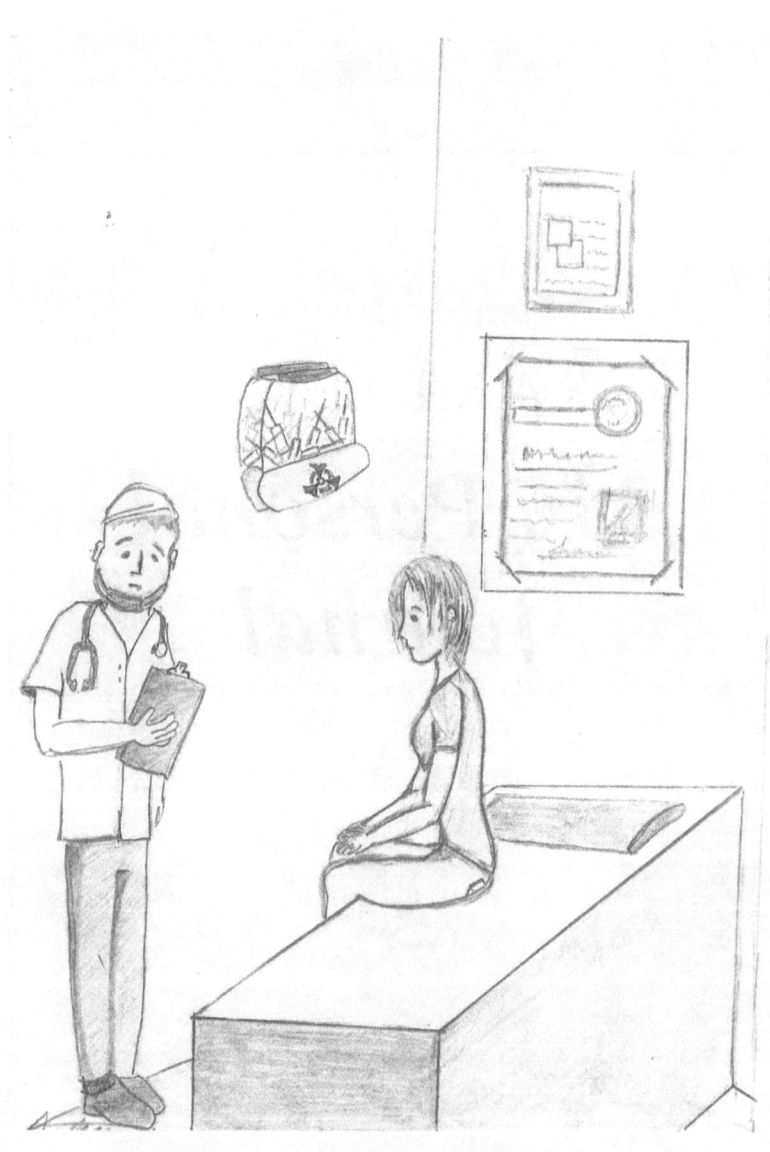

CHAPTER 6

She Said Those Words: "It Is Cancer"

May 12, 2011

As I lay there in a paper gown on the patient table, my mind was focused on the errands I needed to run. I was wishing the doctor would come in so we could get the annual routine physical over with.

It turned out to be anything but routine.

The annual pelvic exam didn't take long, but Dr. W mentioned that the results from my previous ultrasound showed a change in the tissue and recommended a follow up ultrasound.

Slightly concerned, I was still digesting this information as she began the breast exam. We were casually chatting about our summer travel plans when she suddenly hesitated, pausing at an area on my right breast. With apprehension on her face she asked me, "How long has this been here?" Taking my hand, she placed it on the spot so that I could feel it. The lump was palpable and slightly painful when she applied pressure. At that very second my mind froze. I heard her saying that I would need to have some tests done. She added that her office would be calling me to arrange an appointment with the breast specialist. At the checkout desk, I was handed requisitions for a mammogram, breast ultrasound, and uterine ultrasound.

I felt dazed. I do not remember walking to my car, but I do recall just sitting there, forgetting to turn the key. So many thoughts were swirling in my head. I was worried and scared.

I called Marco to tell him what had happened during the appointment. Just needing to hear his voice, I tried to sound like it wasn't a big deal. As soon as I got home, I called my sister, Lynn. She tried to reassure me that it was probably nothing, but I could sense concern in her voice.

It's strange to touch your body and feel something inside that is not supposed to be there. I kept looking at my breast, willing it to be normal and praying the doctor had made a mistake. I didn't want to touch it. Could pressure make it worse or cause it to spread? The mammogram was not until the following Thursday. It was going to be a long week.

May 13, 2011

I've noticed our kids have been asking me, "What's wrong?" and "Are you mad about something?" I must have an angry look on my face. I don't know why I've been so irritated; I don't mean to be critical and moody. I am stopping this today. I need my face to show what is in my heart! I am always so happy to see them come in the door. I need to make sure they know that!

May 16, 2011

I called my friend Myra this morning. We've known each other for twenty years. Myra is clairvoyant, and her intuition is rarely off the mark. Her first words: "I was dreading talking to you today. I have to tell you that your mom is here bringing a message." She continued: "Your mom has tears. It's malignant. Possibly metastasized. You are in a serious place. You can beat this. I don't see you leaving this earth. Add raw foods to your diet. This is not set in stone."

Afterwards I sat there in my bathroom bawling. *This cannot be happening.* I shook my head and heard only, *No, no, no!* in my mind. *I will not accept this!*

In our neighborhood, it is common to see people in golf carts leisurely driving down the streets. Marco and I enjoy taking ours for a ride in the evening after dinner. Tonight, I offered to drive. Slowing to a stop as we approached the cul-de-sac, I said, "I have to talk to you about something." Marco responded with a nervous and hesitant "okay." I relayed my conversation with Myra, blurting out, "She could be wrong, but she believes I have cancer in my breast and possibly my reproductive system too." After a moment of silence I said, "I'm so sorry. I don't want to leave."

The word *cancer* was hard to say out loud; saying the word made it too real. How can this be? I am so healthy, I feel so good. I've been feeling fatigued, but not to the point of thinking something was wrong.

I couldn't even look at Marco. I could taste the pain I was inflicting. I heard his breath catch. He put both arms around me and, with emotion breaking his voice, said, "We will get through this together. We have a lot of traveling to do!" I had to smile. I love him so much. He is the most loving, kind-hearted, selfless, compassionate, and giving person I have ever known. We were both trying to process the situation. I know he is afraid too. It was a silent ride home, both of us struggling with our private thoughts.

May 17, 2011

I called Brooke tonight. She is one of my closest friends, and I wanted to get her input. Living states apart, we spend hours on the phone. Supportive and encouraging, she always knows the right thing to say. I hung up with her feeling as if I just received a big hug!

May 19, 2011

I had my mammogram and breast ultrasound appointments this morning. The technician was professional and pleasant. During the mammogram, we engaged in lighthearted small talk. I wanted to pretend I was somewhere else. When we finished with the mammogram, she headed for the door and said she was going to show the radiologist my films.

When she returned a few minutes later, she relayed, "The radiologist has requested additional positions with the paddles." I knew this was not a good sign. Finally the extra films were completed, and I was ushered into the ultrasound room down the hall.

The ultrasound technician was waiting for me and quickly proceeded with the exam. After our initial greeting, we both remained silent. Then, without any indication of what she had seen, she said, "The radiologist will read both tests, and your doctor should have the results by tomorrow." I left with the uneasy feeling of impending bad news. I'm still not convinced this is really happening to me.

May 23, 2011

Ultrasound with Dr. W at 10:00 a.m.
Breast biopsy with Dr. B at 2:00 p.m.

Results from the mammogram films showed a mass approximately one centimeter in size. The words "We will have to do a biopsy" floated in the air. I had the choice of scheduling it for a later date or doing it right then and there. I opted to get it over with.

The doctor made a quarter-inch incision on the side of my breast and then inserted a core needle four inches through the tissue and into the mass. The machine sounded like a dentist drill. The suction then drew the tissue out, extracting it into a container. She placed a metal marker at the site, which will stay there until surgery. I wasn't informed of that prior to the procedure, and I am not happy about it! If someone is going to leave a foreign object inside your body, they should at least tell you first!

May 27, 2011

Biopsy results with Dr. B at 3:28 p.m.

Diagnosed with breast cancer—HER2+ (human epidermal growth factor receptor 2)

HER2 is a protein that promotes the growth of breast cancer cells; this type of cancer tends to multiply and spread more aggressively than others. Present in about one of every five breast cancers, these cancer cells have a gene mutation that makes an excess of the HER2 protein.

Today I was informed that I definitely have breast cancer. The doctor used the words *invasive* and *aggressive*. I stopped listening after that. Stunned and confused, I got out of there as quickly as I could. The receptionist stopped me, asking me to schedule a follow-up appointment. I couldn't. I couldn't process anything right then. When I got into my car, I saw a missed call from Marco on my phone. He had wanted to come with me today, but I insisted he go to work. He was calling to see how my appointment went. Not ready to say the words, I started to drive home. Feeling disoriented, I realized I wasn't able to focus on driving. Spotting a bank parking lot just ahead, I pulled into an empty space and dialed Marco's number. After telling him the doctor had confirmed that it's cancer, I couldn't find more words. In that moment neither one of us knew what to say. We agreed we would talk when he came home. Our lives may have just changed forever.

I stayed there for a while staring out my windshield, not seeing anything, and not ready to go home. I wanted to be sure I was ready to keep my composure in front of the kids. I didn't want them to worry.

May 28, 2011

Standing in the shower this morning I cried out loud, "I didn't mean it! I didn't mean it!" I was thinking back to that time when thoughts of not wanting to live had crept into my mind.

I don't want to leave! I want to be here with my husband and my kids. I want to see them go to college, get married, have children. I want to be here for them!

When you look your own mortality in the face, everything you thought was important to you changes.

May 29, 2011

Tonight we sat down with James and Leah (our teenagers) to tell them about my diagnosis. We gathered in the living room; they were apprehensive and could sense this was going to be a serious conversation.

I had my words prepared, but when I looked into their eyes, I couldn't speak. With tears swelling, I looked over at Marco and mouthed, "I can't." He graciously began, "Mom had some tests done, and the results confirm that she has breast cancer." The room was still for a moment as the words sunk in. They were both shocked. They were stoic, but the pain was obvious on their faces. We tried to answer their questions and did our best to reassure them. "We will get through this," I said. "Mom will be fine," Marco said. "We will all be fine." I hope it's true. I hate that they have to go through this too.

June 01, 2011

Meeting Dr. H (breast cancer surgeon) at 10:00 a.m.

I wanted to get a second opinion, so we met with Dr. H, a specialist, this morning. A close friend had highly recommended him. He was compassionate and reassuring. I tried not to get emotional, but as he detailed the biopsy results the tears welled up. The diagnosis sounded worse every time I heard it: "Aggressive HER2+." HER2 positive cases constitute only 20 percent of all cases ... lucky me. He added, "A few years ago, we would not have been able to treat this effectively."

The recommended treatments may include surgery, radiation, chemotherapy, and infusions of Herceptin˚, a drug that specifically targets HER2 cells.

This is unbelievable! How did I get this? I'd had the BRACAnalysis˚ genetic test for hereditary breast and ovarian cancer done in June 2007. The results for both genes were negative. I thought I was in the clear.

Today I came across a post by Colette Baron-Reid, an intuitive counselor and accomplished author. The post simply read:

"Listen today ... Answers come from an unexpected source." I'm not exactly keen on the facts I've been given lately; maybe this is a sign that guidance is on the way.

I prayed to the angel of healing. "Archangel Raphael, I need you. Please heal my body."

June 03, 2011

Coincidentally, Eddie Mullins, a spiritual healing strategist and radio show host happened to have Colette Baron-Reid as a guest on his show this morning. She was doing on oracle reading for a woman who had called in, but I truly felt the message spoke to me. She had drawn two cards—the fire prince and the cow. The fire prince card means: Move forward. Be optimistic. Gift of a miracle—healing/facilitator. Connect to your own wholeness. The cow card means: Nourishment. Ask and you will receive blessings.

Ask and you will receive ... okay, God, I'm asking. I could use some help here!

June 06, 2011

MRI scan with contrast at 11:00 a.m.

As I waited for the prick of the IV needle, I wasn't worried about the sting (I didn't even feel it); I was nervous because the doctor had ordered contrast with my MRI, which requires a contrast agent to be injected intravenously. I didn't like the thought of the chemical dye flowing through my veins. I was also concerned about having an allergic reaction.

MRI is an acronym for magnetic resonance imaging. The machine uses a magnetic field and pulses of radio wave energy to take pictures. It can detect structural abnormalities of the body. The contrast dye helps distinguish selected areas from surrounding tissue more clearly.

Zoe, the technician, patiently answered my questions. Her energy was calm and reassuring. After the IV was in place, she led me into the room where the MRI machine stood. I was instructed to lie face down and place my breasts through the holes of a specially designed bolster pad. It seemed weird to leave "the girls" exposed like that. I tried not to think about the cold dye pumping into my veins; it seemed barbaric and wrong. Forty-five minutes later, I heard Zoe announce that we were finished. Whew! I was glad that was done!

During our conversation, Zoe mentioned that she was also a patient of my doctor, and she had gone through this whole "cancer thing" the previous year. She noticed the book I had brought with me: *Living Food Cures* by Joseph R. Farinaccio. We talked about the possibility of a correlation between the food we eat and disease in our bodies. The book shares stories of eleven people who beat disease using raw and whole foods. It turns out that Zoe lives in the same town I live in! We exchanged phone numbers; I really hope to keep in touch. Talking with someone who has gone through all this was encouraging.

June 07, 2011

Will my life ever be the same? Healthy again? In moments of gloom, I wonder if this is the beginning of the end. We've all heard cancer horror stories.

This morning I told Marco, "I don't like being alone anymore. Without distractions, I have to hear my own thoughts."

Yesterday I actually resorted to talking to my breast—to the beast in my breast. "You are not welcome here! You do not have control of my body!"

I have to remember to drink lemon water! Maybe it will help flush out those uninvited cells.

The book *Living Food Cures* poses the question, do I want "life" or "death" at the end of my fork? I've always known that good food is good for you and bad food is bad for you. But now I have good reason to get serious about it. I believe that diet directly affects the immune system and that "dead food" is harmful to my body. Lately I think about everything that goes into my mouth. I'm wondering if it's okay to drink coffee and hoping I can still enjoy a glass of wine.

Found a great quote today: "Acceptance is not submission; it is acknowledgement of the facts of a situation. Then deciding what you're going to do about it" It's by Kathleen Casey Theisen.

June 08, 2011

Purchased a juicing machine today. Excited to try it out!

I recently added Louise Hay's book, *You Can Heal Your Life* to my growing library. It's certainly thought provoking. I believe our thoughts and emotions can manifest illness.

She suggests this positive thought pattern and affirmation: "I lovingly forgive and release all of the past. I choose to fill my world with joy. I love and approve of myself."

I keep finding reminders to love myself, learn forgiveness, and release resentments:

- Find your inner power … and give her a voice.
- You are tougher than you think.
- One day can change the entire course of your life.
- Life is change. Change your perception-change your reality.

I've noticed I'm developing extreme sensitivity to negative energy and conversations. Negativity feels toxic and makes me edgy; I don't want to be around it. Even actors arguing on a television show can be bothersome.

After lots of researching and soul searching, I am definitely leaning toward not doing chemotherapy treatment. I'm thinking the potential harm is not worth the benefit in my case. Chemo treatment is palliative (not expected to cure the patient), not curative. In some cases it is administered simply in the hope of prolonging the patient's life. The drugs seek and destroy cancer cells, but also kill healthy cells as well. Some chemotherapy medications are so potent and toxic that the patient can develop second cancers such as leukemia. Chemo drugs are known to damage the liver and to affect the brain, nervous system, and most all other organs. If it isn't toxic, why do the nurses wear protective gear when they administer it?

CHAPTER 7

This Just Got Real: Waiting Rooms, Exam Rooms, and Operating Rooms

June 09, 2011

Oncologist appointment with Dr. C at 8:30 a.m.

Marco insisted on being with me for my appointment. Thank God! Just having him by my side makes me stronger. I could not believe I was walking into the cancer institute as a patient. I have driven by that building countless times, never considering that one day I could be on the inside looking out. Sitting there in the crowded waiting room felt surreal. I still can't believe my body is doing this! On the way back to the exam room, I had to stop and give a "donation." They needed a blood draw for labs, which include cancer marker tests (CA15-3, CEA).

Dr. C was cordial and knowledgeable. I was told she is highly regarded by her peers.

I found it interesting that cancer is so complex. The fundamental biology of a cancer cell can vary greatly. There are many variants in a breast cancer diagnosis. The pathology can be HER2 positive/negative, estrogen positive/negative, progesterone positive/negative, invasive/noninvasive, and numerous combinations.

Although my cancer type is highly aggressive, I was told that my prognosis is excellent. The recommended treatment protocol includes:

- Chemotherapy (taxol)
- Herceptin
- Breast surgery
- Radiation (possibly)

Surgery options are lumpectomy and mastectomy. If I choose lumpectomy, I will require radiation as well. If I choose mastectomy, no radiation will be necessary.

The oncologist was looking at my recent mammogram films comparing them to my films from the previous year when she noticed that the mass area had been present in my films from last year! It had not been caught by the human eyes of the radiologist and had never been flagged! *What?*

Displaying the films, she pointed out the same spot in both films, but a white ring surrounding the tumor was visible in the new films; new computer technology had detected and circled the area of the mass. Learning that this beast has been in my body all this time was shattering! I felt a rush of anger and then disbelief! Why had the mass been overlooked? If we had known then, it would have been smaller; I could be looking at an entirely different scenario.

Dr. C conveyed that clinical observations point to stage one.

Some cells on the muscle will need to be scraped off, and indications are that it has not spread to the lymph nodes. That is definitely good news!

When I voiced my hesitation about doing chemo, she said, "You can compromise with me, but you cannot compromise with cancer."

As we talked about my diagnosis and prognosis, she wrote everything out longhand on a sheet of paper for me. I am grateful for that. I would not have absorbed it all.

When we finished with the oncologist, I met with a gene research specialist to discuss the BRACAnalysis genetic test for hereditary breast and ovarian cancer. I told her that I'd had the gene test when my sister was diagnosed a few years ago, and it was negative. She said the testing is more extensive now than it was a few years ago. I am not interested in doing it again.

As we were getting into the car, I remembered that I hadn't mentioned the metal taste I have in my mouth. I had also meant to ask if there are any clinical trials for which I could be a candidate. I'm definitely taking my notepad with me from now on!

June 10, 2011

I'm finding that people feel compelled to give their opinion on my treatment quandary. I've gotten mixed reactions when they hear I am contemplating not doing chemotherapy. Most are surprised when I say I'm looking into alternative and natural healing methods.

Some have said, "You have to do chemo—it's the only way to cure this!" I know they mean well, but I'm not convinced that's the best course of action for me. Would they be as quick to dive in if their bodies were the ones being poisoned? It is my body, and I will decide what I will allow to be done to it!

This morning, a like-minded friend called me and asked, "Have you considered holistic methods?" It was so refreshing—and validating—to talk to someone who shares the idea that it is at least worth considering.

Some years ago, I injured my back while lifting boxes. My L5-S1 disk was herniated. There was almost zero tissue between the vertebrae. It was very debilitating, and even slight movements could cause sudden, excruciating pain. Three different doctors told me I would need spinal fusion surgery. At the first doctor visit, I overheard the doctor laughingly tell the patient in the next room, "I just bought a new boat. Now I have to figure out how to pay for it." A few minutes later he was in my room telling me I have one of the worst cases he has ever seen, and my only option was major surgery. Hoping for a different prognosis, I sought second, third, and fourth opinions. Two more doctors echoed the same recommendation. The fourth doctor was willing to help me avoid it. Wanting to exhaust every other action before succumbing to surgery, I did physical therapy, acupuncture, DRX9000 chiropractic treatments, yoga, Reiki healing, essential oil therapy, and more. I kept Archangel Raphael on speed dial. I no longer have that pain. I can run and lift weights again. If it starts to feel irritated, I just take it easy for a couple days. I am so thankful for that fourth doctor who was willing to think outside the box and explore alternative methods.

Tonight I found my daughter lying on her bed crying. When I asked her what was the matter, she spoke through her tears, "I don't want you to be sick." I know my son is stressed too; today he hugged me and said, "I am here for you. I know this is hard."

I don't like seeing them upset, especially when I know it's because of me.

June 11, 2011

Practiced a Louise Hay healing meditation this morning:

Envision a green light … a pinpoint pulsating in your heart growing outward, then throughout the whole body to others and other things. Repeat the affirmation, "With every breath I take, I am getting healthier."

I need to remember to take deep cleansing breaths for more oxygen instead of short, shallow breaths.

What we give out comes back to us, multiplied.

June 12, 2011

Not such a good day. I was tense all day, and I could see that Marco was edgy too. I know that this cancer crap doesn't just affect me; it affects the whole family.

Marco and I somehow got into a conversation about the fact that I don't want to do chemo, and he expressed that he didn't like—or wasn't necessarily in agreement with—my attitude toward my doctor. Maybe I had said "I feel like a science project" too many times. Maybe "science project" isn't the best analogy, but I feel as if I have lost control over my own body.

Typically, I am a positive-minded person; I don't like feeling negative and resentful. So, why do I feel this anger? Why did this happen? I am irritated that my body has let me down.

Every doctor's visit and every barbaric test feels like an assault to my body. Upon entering an examination room, I automatically step into defense mode. I don't want anyone to touch me.

Marco is annoyed with my moodiness. I sense he is feeling helpless because he is unable to fix this, and he is frustrated. We ended up in a fight. He snapped at me to stop acting like a martyr. I was instantly angry and hurt at the same time and shouted at him to just leave me alone. I could see the regret on his face, as he was instantly sorry those words had spilled out. He abruptly left the bedroom and closed the door behind him. Collapsing on the bed, I curled up beneath the covers. When my pity party ended, I found the motivation to make my way to the laundry room. There were clothes that needed to go in the dryer, and I need a reason to get out of bed. As soon as I entered the laundry room, Marco was behind me wrapping his arms around my waist. He held me tight as he said, "I'm so sorry. This is bad. I didn't mean it. We can't let this divide us." I could hear anguish in his voice. I was reminded why I love him so much and how he makes me feel so safe.

I told him I have no intention of sticking around just to be sick for the rest of my life, to become a burden. Then, knowing I shouldn't say it, I did: "Maybe this is my time. Maybe I am supposed to go this way." Choking back tears he whispered, "No, no. Don't say that." That was the first time I have spoken those words. It will also be the last.

I consider myself to be a strong person; I kick ass when I need to. I've always moved full speed ahead and not looked back. Now I feel emotionally fragile and afraid I will crumble into pieces. It is scary not knowing what lies ahead. Some days it would be easier to just stay in bed and pretend this isn't happening. This is one "adventure" I would rather avoid.

On Facebook this morning, I saw a message from a British friend who had been a crewmember on my first ship. He was just checking in to say hello and let me know he had been in touch with our mutual friend in Hawaii. He doesn't know about my diagnosis and has no idea how much his sweet note meant to me. Happy memories of those days brightened my mood and made me forget for a few minutes that I have cancer.

June 13, 2011

I want to be happy again. I am angry way too often. Now I feel as if I'm putting my family on edge. I have to stop being so moody. The kids are spending more time at friends' houses. I am nitpicking and over-mothering. Maybe I'm afraid to find out that they don't need me as they used to.

In preparation for my PET test (positron emission tomography scan) tomorrow, I cannot eat or drink anything that contains carbohydrates or sugar for a minimum of twenty-four hours prior to the scan. It's important that my glucose level is low when we begin the procedure. Avoiding sugar is not easy—it's in almost everything! I had to do my homework. I was surprised to discover restaurants commonly add sugar to dishes you would never expect to contain sugar. Not cool!

I have read that cancer cells love sugar. Breast tissue contains insulin receptors, and insulin is a stimulant of cell growth. I'm thinking that pumping sugar solution into my veins may not be the best plan.

June 15, 2011

PET scan 8:00 a.m.

I weighed myself this morning. I've lost eight pounds since my diagnosis, most likely because I am more conscious about what goes into my mouth. Love my juicer!

I was apprehensive about having the PET scan. The evaluation determines whether or not cancer cells have spread to other parts of the body. When I arrived, the technician immediately put me at ease with his warm smile. He guided me to a small room where there was a huge reclining chair. As I settled in, I noticed the IV start kit on the table.

First he tested my blood sugar level by pricking my finger. It was seventy-one, which is low. That was followed with an intravenous fusion of a saline-sugar solution, and finally the radioactive fluid was attached to my IV.

The worst part of all this was thinking about the radioactive solution flowing into my body.

The technician kindly offered me a warm blanket and told me I could rest for about forty-five minutes. The chair was super comfy, but relax? I don't think so! When he returned, we walked to the computerized axial tomography (CAT) scan room.

I was instructed to lie on my back with my arms extended up above my head. I was to breathe normally. (Yeah, right.) I closed my eyes and tried to focus on calming thoughts. The table began to slide back and forth like a two-way toboggan. About fifteen minutes later, I heard the technician declare, "Okay, you are all finished." As

I was leaving, he gently added, "You have the best doctor for your type of cancer."

I was cautioned not to let the radioactive fluid sit in the bladder. It is important to drink *lots* of water to purge it out through the urine. Bottoms up! Apparently you can be radioactive for six to ten hours post procedure. I believe it, because even my poo smelled nuclear. They also advised me not to pass through airport security, as the radiation could set off an alarm in the radiation detection equipment. Additionally, I was told to flush the toilet twice after voiding, and to stay away from small children and anyone with a compromised immune system. My god, what is this stuff?

Marco and I decided it would be best if I stayed at a hotel that night, since our son had just had oral surgery.

I ordered a pizza, took an Epson salt bath, meditated, balanced my chakras, and did a Reiki healing treatment. Then I went for a long walk on the beach. Looking at the sea and feeling the foamy waves on my ankles, I silently prayed: *God, please give me the courage and strength to make the right decisions about my treatment.*

It was a long night. I didn't want to be alone. I thought about how thankful I was to have my husband and children in my life.

"There are always flowers for those who want to see them." —Henri Matisse

Calming Meditation:

Sit quietly, close your eyes, and allow your attention to gently focus on your breathing.
On your in breath, think: "I am …"
On your out breath, think: "… at peace."

June 16, 2011

Appointment with plastic surgeon at 10:00 a.m.

We met Dr. S today. I really liked him. Besides having an excellent reputation, he was confident and kindhearted. We discussed the pros and cons of a mastectomy and a lumpectomy.

I'm leaning toward having a bi-lateral mastectomy. If I go with the mastectomy, I won't require radiation. I would rather go ahead and remove both breasts so I don't have to worry about the possibility of going through this again with the other one. Besides I want them to look alike—comparing apples to apples—as opposed to doing one now and potentially the other one another time.

Unfortunately, Dr. S is almost certain that he won't be able to preserve my nipples due to the fact that I had a mastopexy (breast lift) with augmentation fifteen years ago. The scars from that procedure (though barely visible) will prevent the tissue from surviving without blood supply from underlying tissue. That was hard to hear. I don't want to lose my nipples. *What will my breasts look like? Will I be disfigured? What about sexual sensation?*

Today I heard from a friend who told me about a holistic physician who practices Oriental medicine and acupuncture. He is on staff at the hospital where I will have surgery, and he provides acupuncture to patients during procedures in the operating room.

Hmm … didn't I just ask the universe for knowledge and direction?

I once had an acupuncture treatment in Japan; the doctor was blind but knew exactly where to place the needles. It was astonishing, and I felt revitalized!

June 19, 2011

We hosted a Father's Day BBQ with family and a few neighbors today. We had a great time! James and Leah made Marco's day with homemade cards that contained handwritten words of love and appreciation that stirred his emotions They made him feel so loved and proud of them.

The festivities were therapeutic and helped us put aside our situation for the day.

June 20, 2011

Acupuncture appointment at 9:00 a.m.

I met Dr. N today and had an acupuncture treatment. He is proficient in Traditional Chinese Medicine and explained the benefits of acupuncture therapy. His genuine caring manner put me at ease right away. He also recommended daily juicing and supplements.

Acupuncture boosts your immune system and can treat countless conditions, from relieving stress to managing pain. The procedure was painless and, surprisingly, very relaxing. He started the session with a short massage, and then gently inserted the needles at various points on my body. Once the needles were in place, he applied heat and essential oils. With so many "assaults" (tests/exams/labs) on my body, it felt good to do something kind to it!

June 21, 2011

I have an appointment with the oncologist to get the results of my labs this afternoon (PET scans, CA125, and blood tests)

I am so nervous, I cannot think or concentrate on anything.

I prayed: "Dear God, Archangel Raphael, Archangel Michael, Reiki Masters, and Guides too, please let me get good news today. I want to hear the cancer is localized in the breast only and is not anywhere else. Thank you in advance for restored health."

And so it is!

The PET scan confirmed that the cancer has not spread to other areas of my body; it has *not* metastasized! Blood work labs were all normal, including CA125 for ovaries. We are so relieved! Finally some good news!

Maybe some divine intervention has stopped this cancer beast in its tracks.

"Never, never, never, never give up!" – Winston Churchill

"What lies behind us and what lies before us are small matters compared to what lies within us." —Ralph Waldo Emerson

June 23, 2011

I can't believe the first available date for surgery is July 13, almost two months after my diagnosis. This waiting sucks!

It's getting frustrating—all the testing, waiting for results, scheduling endless appointments.

June 27, 2011

Appointment with a certified clinical nutritionist at 3:00 p.m.

More blood draws—will I have any left after all this? Blood Sugar is 140.

The nutritionist recommended I start a detox regimen, and begin taking active nattokinase enzyme (Advanced Natto Formula), prenatal vitamins because they are more potent, and alkaline drops (added to drinking water).

It was interesting to learn that every human being has potential cancer cells in his or her body. The unhealthy cells either flush out or become rogue cells that are capable of organizing a tumor party. A strong immune system helps to destroy the defective cells.

June 29, 2011

I had a Pranic healing session with Charles this morning; he is a clairvoyant medical intuitive. He's amazing, and his insight is spot on! Pranic healing is a health-restoring method that uses Prana (life energy) to heal ailments in the body by manipulating the person's energy field, removing blockages, and infusing the body with healing energy. It astonishes me that he can do this over the phone, but without a doubt, it has eliminated issues for me in the past.

June 30, 2011

Acupuncture treatment at 2:00 p.m.

While talking with our family friend Lula, I found out that Dr. N is a friend of hers and she highly recommends him! Is it a small world or is this synchronicity?

He is producing a video on the holistic approach to disease and asked if I would consider being interviewed for it. I told him I would think about it. I agree the message needs to get out there. In addition to mainstream medications and surgical procedures, there are holistic and complementary therapies that provide further options.

Holistic practitioners believe that imbalance (physical, emotional, or spiritual) in a person's life can have a negative affect on overall health. Holistic principles involve fixing the cause of the condition, not just alleviating the symptoms. The patient is a person, not a disease.

Integrative medicine unites conventional medicine with alternative therapies, using the best of both worlds to achieve optimal health.

July 1, 2011

Appointment with Dr. H at 8:00 a.m.

He was very considerate and made me feel as if I was the only patient he had today. He spent so much time with me and didn't leave the room before pausing to ask if I had any more questions he could answer. Taking my hand in his, he told me he was sorry I am going through this; it was genuine and heartfelt.

We discussed:

- Tramadol vs. morphine (I will have both. Tramadol does not suppress the immune system as morphine can.)
- Going home with drains in the incisions post surgery
- Scraping of cancer cells if present on the muscle
- Removing the lymph node and biopsy of lymph nodes
- Hospital stay and recovery period
- Permission for Dr. K to be in the operating room
- My allergy to adhesive bandages and tape
- Nipple preservation—unlikely

July 4, 2011

We took the boat out for a while today—perfect for unwinding! We visited Peck Lake and took a walk on the beach. Feeling introspective, I reflected on pivotal points in my life—losing my mom, leaving Nebraska to travel, getting married, having children. It is fascinating how our choices, which can seem small, set major things in motion and chart our course.

July 5, 2011

Zoe, the MRI technician, and I met for dinner tonight. We had a great conversation and discovered we have a lot in common. It's crazy to think we met because of cancer, but I think we will become good friends! When I shared my concern about how "they" will look afterward, she graciously offered to let me see "hers." We had a good laugh, but what she didn't know, was how comforting that was for me—they looked great!

July 6, 2011

Appointment with Nutritionist at 9:00 a.m.

I had an ionic footbath this morning. Not sure I'm believing this actually works. Then I came home with seven more bottles of cancer-fighting supplements—ugh!

Acupuncture appointment with Dr. N at 3:00 p.m.

He asked if I would be willing to be interviewed on camera for a segment about holistic treatments for cancer. Interviews would take place in his office, in the operating room prior to surgery, at the hospital, and again during my treatment afterwards. At first I said yes, but now after coming home and thinking about it, I'm not sure I want to do the video. I feel stressed about it and not sure I am comfortable with the exposure.

I had a tough day today. Surgery day is inching closer. I am feeling unsure of which "experts" to listen to and wondering if the nutritionist is right or wrong. She tried to talk me out of having the mastectomy surgery.

I feel that oncologists push pharmaceuticals, and now the nutritionist is pushing supplements. I have ten bottles of supplements already sitting on my counter and today she added coral calcium, melatonin, curcumin, rubidium, vitamin D, and cesium.

I find myself resenting that other people don't have to alter their diets and their lives. I even sometimes envy my family and friends.

I'm questioning Western medicine endorsements for toxic cancer treatments; does chemotherapy do more harm than good? Patients are not always told the treatment is considered palliative not curative.

I've been reading about alternative treatments. There is some wild stuff out there! Apparently coffee enemas help to detoxify the body. I'm quite open-minded, but I think I will pass on that one!

July 7, 2011

Appointment with Dr. S at noon

Marco met me at the plastic surgeon's office, and I completed the required paperwork. I noticed the procedure stated augmentation with silicone implants, not saline. When I pointed it out to the receptionist, she quickly corrected it. I definitely want to stay with saline.

Dr. S was patient and answered all my questions. We discussed that I would like my breasts to be the same size afterwards. I do not want them bigger. In hopes of avoiding a second procedure, I told him I would rather have them smaller if increasing size would require me to have a tissue expander. A tissue expander is an expandable balloon implanted temporarily under the skin. Over a period of weeks or months, a saline solution is injected to slowly stretch the overlaying skin. A second procedure is required to replace the expander with the permanent breast implant.

I'm hoping it doesn't come to that. I asked if the breast would feel heavier due to replacing tissue with the implant, and he said it's not likely. Dr. S confirmed that it won't be possible to save my nipples due to the scar pattern from my previous mastopexy. He mentioned that I could do a procedure later on that creates a nipple by twisting the skin and then tattooing an areola. I know he was trying to be positive, but the thought of it made me feel sick to my stomach.

Leah wanted me to ask the doctor if I would still have "our freckles." I explained that we both have the exact same two freckles in the exact same place on the left breast. He assured me the freckles can stay. That will make her smile!

Surgery is less than a week away. They expect the procedure to take five to six hours (two and a half to three hours for each doctor).

I reminded the medical assistant about my allergy to tape/bandage adhesives. She went over the pre- and post-op requirements and limitations with me.

They have arranged for home nurse visits to change the bandages and drains.

Marco asked me if I wanted to lie down with him and cuddle. How does he just know when I need him? My right breast and armpit are quite sore today. Not sure why.

I've been a mess the last two days. I'm wondering if it's due to detoxification treatments, acupuncture, or is it just because surgery day is right around the corner.

I called Dr. N to let him know that, after giving it more thought, I've decided I'm not comfortable with sharing my story on camera. He was understanding and told me not to worry about it.

I need to keep this journey personal right now, without adding more stress. Most days I can be optimistic and deal with it; but sometimes the reality of it takes my breath away.

Explored more research on treatments, side effects, and alternatives today; separating factual information from marketing hype can be tricky.

July 8, 2011

Hospital pre-op appointment at 9:00 a.m.

First I answered a bazillion questions. Then I filled out forms and more forms. The anesthesiologist stopped by to introduce himself and asked if I had any questions. What questions should I have? Will you make sure I continue to breathe?

Next on the agenda was an EKG and a blood draw. The doctor's order included tests for potassium and various chemicals. What chemicals?

If one more person tells me I have to remove my belly button ring prior to surgery I will scream. I *know* already!

This is all starting to feel too real. I'm still experiencing discomfort and pain in my right breast. It feels as if the metal marker left behind during the biopsy has moved and is poking me. It has been there a long time—almost three weeks! I want it out of me!

Dr. H called this evening to ask if I would be willing to give a small portion of my cancer tissue to the hospital for cancer research. He said he wanted to call me personally before the center contacted me.

I told him my only concern was that he have enough for my pathology testing. He said, "There will be enough for everyone." That made me laugh! It is strange to think about someone wanting my tissue. He asked how I was doing and expressed regret that the nipples cannot be saved. I was touched by his empathy.

CHAPTER 8

What Are My Surgery Options?

July 10, 2011

I took a bath in Epson salt to relax and clear any toxins. Sitting there in the warm water, I held my breasts, touching them, mourning their imminent loss. I have to keep this in perspective. I am not losing an arm or a leg. They are just boobs.

I shaved my legs and underarms for the last time before surgery. I was told to do it three days prior as the doctors do not want any risk of open cuts or scrapes that could become infected.

July 11, 2011

Acupuncture at 11:00 a.m.

As I was getting ready to leave, I started telling Dr. N how reassuring it was to know he would be with me in the operating room. Then, halfway through my words, the tears started. He put his arms out, gave me a warm hug, and said, "I wondered when you were going to do that."

He proceeded to tell me that another patient—one he wouldn't expect to—cried at every treatment. Apparently the acupuncture can facilitate emotional release. (Maybe that's why I've been in crazy town!)

A package came in the mail this morning. It was beautifully wrapped and contained journals, a pen, and two pairs of organic Alpaca fleece socks. It was from our friend Mari. She is an animal advocate and the most eco-friendly person I know, and she assured me that the alpacas are just sheared and not harmed. The socks truly feel like heaven on my feet!

The phone has been ringing nonstop, and I feel so loved. It is hard for people to know what to say. Just taking the time to call means so much.

I've been busy trying to get things done before surgery. Even cleaning the house is a welcome distraction. I scheduled the dishwasher repair, arranged the furniture donation, ordered Leah's birthday cake, and confirmed doctor's appointments.

The representative from the cancer research center called to explain that they would like to acquire some tissue samples, both normal and cancerous, for some trials they are working on with Scripps Research Institute. I feel I should do this, and agreed to sign the papers in pre-op on the morning of my surgery. Maybe it will further research and help in some way. It was so weird to get a call from a stranger asking to have part of my body!

I checked out the website regarding nipple tattooing that I heard about. It looks interesting. Maybe it will be an option at some point. They are 3-D tattoos, and they look fairly realistic.

I am worried what my husband's reaction to the new me will be. Every time I bring it up, he assures me that it won't matter. I asked him to feel the lump tonight. He didn't really want to, but I needed him to.

Actually, the lump feels different than it did two months ago. It used to feel smooth and soft; now it is hard and bumpy. Maybe it is dying!

July 12, 2011

Tomorrow is surgery day.

I don't feel nervous; I just feel sad—sad that my family has to go through this, sad that I have to go through this, and sad that my body will be forever changed.

The kids have been so positive and brave. Leah has asked a lot of questions. James gives me lots of hugs. I hope they are okay. I know Marco is worried, but he is trying to stay strong for me.

I am just ready to get this over with. It's 11:00 p.m. I'm taking "the girls" to bed for the last time.

July 13, 2011

Surgery day: bilateral mastectomy with reconstruction

The alarm sounded at 4:30 a.m.

I zombie walked into the shower and washed with antibacterial soap to alleviate any skin bacteria. Staring at the clothes in my closet, I chose a button-down blouse and leggings. We are supposed to arrive at the hospital by 6:30. Surgery is scheduled at 8:00.

Good-bye, boobies … good-bye, nipples …

Good riddance "C" word!

It can't hurt to throw in a positive affirmation: I am completely at peace, knowing I have healing energy around me.

I am completely at peace ... (wish I felt what my lips are saying).

Well, it's time to go to the hospital. Let's get this over with!

After a thirty-minute drive, we arrived at the hospital and checked in at the reception desk. The representative from the cancer research center brought me papers to sign, giving the authorization for them to receive the tissue—my tissue. I reminded myself it could benefit other women. She told us that they have had success with RNA injected into guppies. It kills the cancer cells but not the surrounding tissue. Why doesn't the public hear more about these strides in research?

A smiling nurse escorted me to the pre-op room. She presented me with a stylish (sarcasm) gown, and I quickly changed. As soon as I settled onto the bed, someone was there to start the IV. Zoe stopped by to say hello and give me a hug. Dr. H and Dr. S both popped in briefly on their way to the operating room. Dr. N arrived and placed a few acupuncture points to relax me. The last thing I remember is one of the nurses saying, "I'm going to give you a cocktail."

I awoke in recovery to the sound of the acupuncturist's voice. I smiled and drifted back to sleep. I vaguely remember my bed being maneuvered into my hospital room.

Leah sweetly offered to spend the night in the hospital with me. I was so grateful to have her by my side. Not sure how much sleep she got in that recliner though! James was working and came with Marco in the morning.

Waking up during the night, I was itching everywhere! I remember frantically telling the nurse, "I told them I was allergic to bandage adhesives!" She promptly removed the bandages and replaced them with Ace wraps.

The itching could also have been from the morphine, the prep solution, or antibiotic, but she wasn't taking any chances. The Benadryl* injected into my IV finally brought some relief. The next morning when my doctors arrived, I learned that there had been some issues during surgery.

The isotope fluid would not flow to the lymph nodes, so Dr. H, the cancer surgeon, could not locate which ones were the sentinel nodes. He determined it was necessary to remove ten lymph nodes. I was not happy about this because the more nodes removed, the more likely the patient is to have edema and lymphatic complications.

The plastic surgeon, Dr. S, told me that the right breast procedure went well; there were no problems with the implant insertion. But there were issues with the left breast. When the implant was inserted, the bottom left quadrant of skin turned blue, indicating a high risk of skin dying due to lack of blood. This was probably a result of existing scar tissue from my previous mastopexy cutting off the blood supply. So he had no choice but to remove the implant and insert an expander (exactly what I had hoped to avoid).

I was expecting to wake up with two new breasts; now I am lopsided. Saying I am disappointed is an understatement. However, I am thankful that Dr. S had the knowledge and skill to make the right call during surgery. I know this will mean a long process of expansion appointments and then additional surgery, followed by another recovery period.

I have to keep reminding myself that the important thing is they removed the cancer. It is out of my body! Gone!

July 14, 2011

James came to the hospital today. It was so good to (carefully) hug him.

When Dr. H stopped by, I asked him if the tumor had appeared bumpy, and he confirmed that it had. I was intrigued that, initially, it had felt smooth to the touch, but just a few weeks later, the texture had changed, and from the outside, it felt bumpy to the touch. He remarked that it could be that it was healing from the biopsy (but that was six weeks ago). I prefer to believe it was healing, as in dying, due to all the alternative treatments.

I have no doubt that acupuncture helped to keep the cancer from growing and spreading.

I slept most of the day. Leah spent the night with me again. She will be happy to say good-bye to that recliner.

Dr. N came to my hospital room and gave me an acupuncture treatment. My plastic surgeon stopped in and rewrapped the ace bandage.

July 15, 2011

Both surgeons agreed to discharge me. I left the hospital before noon.

Feels good to be home!

- Rash still itchy; took more Benadryl.
- Very sore today; it's painful to move, especially when getting up or sitting down.
- Much more discomfort in the breast with the expander than the breast with the implant.
- Have a drain tube in each breast (ugh!).
- Slept most of the afternoon.

I am not looking forward to two weeks of trying to sleep propped up in a sitting position!

July 17, 2011

I didn't take any pain medication before going to bed—big mistake! Woke up at 3:30 a.m. and took acetaminophen. I didn't need anything for pain the rest of the day.

Rash is very itchy and irritating, especially under both arms where the tape was.

Went out for a short walk with my husband; felt so good to breathe fresh air and absorb the sunshine.

Removed the Ace bandage; it was loose anyway and bothering me.

Saw my incisions—it was shocking and made me sad. Left one flat, and right one looks half the size it was. I cried.

July 19, 2011

Nausea/vomiting
Diarrhea

Weakness
Discomfort from expander

Dr. R called with post-op pathology results; they are excellent! All margins surrounding tumor are clear! All skin areas are clear! All lymph nodes are clear! Left breast is clear! Tumor measured 2.2 centimeters (determined stage 2 due to size).

July 20, 2011

Nausea/Diarrhea

First shower … first time seeing myself naked. I started sobbing, afraid I will never feel sexy again. I am cut from one side to the other—incisions all the way across both breasts and another one under right arm/lymph node area.

Leah overheard me and came in to ask if I was okay. I feel bad that she heard my tantrum. When Marco got home we talked about it; he sweetly reminded me to stay focused on defeating the cancer.

July 21, 2011

Appointment with plastic surgeon at 2:00 p.m.

Drains came out today—yay! I felt a stinging sensation as they were being pulled out of my body. I closed my eyes, but Marco told me he could not believe how long they were (maybe five inches).

The medical assistant told me I can stop taking the oral antibiotic today.

July 24, 2011

Took first post-op pictures today. Eleven days since surgery. I want to see the changes and how the healing progresses.

What a shockwave every time I get a glimpse of myself in the mirror. I am mad that I had to do this to my body.

July 25, 2011

Swelling subsiding. I am not happy with size of the implant; it is smaller than I expected. Hard to find tops that camouflage "One-Boobie Bree".

July 26, 2011

Acupuncture appointment at 1:00 p.m.

Drove myself to my appointment—first time driving post surgery. Told him about pain in my middle back due to sleeping (at least trying to sleep) sitting up for the last two weeks. He had me lie on my side while he placed needles on either side of my spine. Voila! Already feels better!

July 27, 2011

Back muscle tension completely gone. I'm having significant pain in the left breast due to the expander. Not only can I feel it, I can actually see where it is poking me. So weird.

Leah and I took a drive to the beach and went for a long walk. Being by the ocean with the sand in my toes and the sun on my face helped me to reboot. Awesome time—I'm feeling blessed.

Tonight still having discomfort around the expander. I wonder if driving yesterday irritated the muscle. Maybe I was too active?

July 28, 2011

Appointment with Dr. H (surgeon) at 3:00 p.m.
Appointment with Dr. S (plastic surgeon) at 4:15 p.m.

Dr. H went over the pathology report details again. My prognosis looks good. He brought up that lymphedema is a possibility, but that doesn't mean it will happen.

They say it is important to remember not to take blood pressure or blood draws on my right arm—not ever! It could trigger lymphedema, a condition that can be a result of lymph node removal. Lymphedema is the buildup of fluid, which causes localized swelling in the arms. It can appear in some people months or years after treatment.

We touched on additional treatments (chemotherapy/Herceptin infusions) that may be required. I mentioned my concern about the long-term effects of those medications.

Today is my first expansion procedure with Dr. S. It was a strange sensation—like pumping up a tire, but the tire is inside of you. A magnet at the end of the tube located the port and marked the spot with an "x." The needle was then inserted, and saline was pumped into the expander implant. No pain, just pressure. It actually felt a little better afterwards.

I told Dr. D that the right breast is half the size it was, adding that I may want a larger size. He said not a problem. He will tell me when we are at the point where final size is pretty much established, and then I can make that call.

Feeling grateful to have doctors who sincerely care. Dr. D answers all my questions and never makes me feel rushed.

July 29, 2011

We had Leah's "sweet sixteen" celebration tonight at Taverna Opa, a Greek restaurant. I made the mistake of having a cocktail in a restaurant that actually encourages you to dance on the tables ... *Opa!*

July 30, 2011

Lesson learned ... dancing two weeks post-op may not have been the best idea! Feeling it today!

August 9, 2011

Acupuncture at 9:30 a.m.
Appointment with an intuitive healer at 2:15 p.m.

Mentioned I was having pain/tightness under my right arm. Dr. N placed a needle and hit it right on. I know because I felt a slight pain and the release. Felt immediate relief.

Out of curiosity, I met with a medical intuitive today. She claims to rely on her intuitive guidance and insight to find the root cause of a physical or emotional condition. I already know intuition is a powerful tool. Why not see what she has to say?

She shuffled the deck of oracle cards and then fanned them face down on the table. I was then invited to choose one. Turning over my card of choice, I noticed that beneath the picture were the words *Healing—second chance.*

Explaining the message, she said, "It means you defeated it, but it is up to you to do the work." I had not told her what my health issue was. She then asked me to stand up with my arms straight out and palms facing upward. Scanning my body with energy clearing disks, she stated that she was not picking up blockages, but was getting breast issues. Coincidence?

August 10, 2011

Meeting with the nutritionist at 10:00 a.m.

The nutritionist had insisted on doing a microscopic hair strand analysis. I wasn't impressed or even convinced of the results. Her disclaimers didn't exactly lend credibility to the outcome (for example, hair color can taint the results).

I returned a few bottles of unopened supplements, explaining that I know myself and know that I will not comply with swallowing thirty to fifty pills per day. She was obviously agitated with my stand on things. I relayed to her that I had come to her for nutritional advice, not just to replace convention pharmaceuticals with herbal supplements. She had recommended more supplements during each of my visits, and the cost had really been adding up.

As I was about to leave she pitched, "Maybe next time you will let me do the iconic foot bath." (I'm not sure there will be a next time.) After I paid for today's charges, her sarcastic remark was, "I hope your acupuncturist can help you."

August 12, 2011

Appointment with oncologist at 10:30 a.m.

Arrived at the office only to be told that they did not have me on the schedule. My appointment had been "lost." Little did I know that would entail a three-hour wait.

When the nurse practitioner finally came into the room, she was asking questions that had obvious answers, and this annoyed me (or maybe I'm just angry at the world). As she finished typing my answers into the computer, she stood up, approached me, and reached to open the paper gown. "I'm just going to take a peak." I snapped "No!" She looked surprised and questioned, "No?" I pulled the gown closed and replied, "No, I'd rather not." Looking perplexed, she turned and left the room.

I glanced over at Marco. He was staring down at the floor and looked really uncomfortable. The room filled with awkward silence.

We went today expecting to be told the treatment plan would include chemotherapy. That was confirmed when we finally met with Dr. C. The oncologist informed us that the recommended treatment includes taxol (a chemotherapy drug), as well as Herceptin infusions. Herceptin is a target therapy drug recommended for HER2 positive cancers.

The oncologist said I have the worst kind of breast cancer. I wish everyone would stop saying that.

Statistically, I have a 35 percent chance of recurrence with no adjunctive treatment (chemo/Herceptin) and a 5 percent chance of recurrence with adjunctive treatment. So my take-away is that two out of three women do not need adjunctive therapy!

I am not convinced that I need to do this to save my life. I asked, "Can you tell me that chemotherapy would cure my cancer?" She could not.

I conveyed that I am having a hard time understanding why chemotherapy and Herceptin infusions are necessary with negative lymph node involvement, clear margins, clear left breast, and the bi-lateral mastectomy.

The constant response to my enquiry was, "It is the recommended protocol." I had been informed from the beginning that surgery is only the first step. With my pathology profile, adjunctive therapy would be compulsory. I was ambivalent and wanted a better explanation. Being told, "because it is protocol" sounded just like my dad saying "because I said so."

Dr. C said she would like me to meet with a doctor in Miami who has done a lot research with Herceptin. In the meantime, she will retest the HER2 pathology just to reconfirm.

Someone from the medical center physical therapy department called today. My first reaction was that I don't need physical therapy; but now I'm thinking it might be a good idea. I want to hear what they have to say about lymphedema prevention and range of motion.

It is getting late; I should be in bed. But here I sit, thinking about this lymphatic matter. I'm wondering how cancer cells could travel to lymph nodes if the isotope solution wasn't able to find a path. I'm not happy that ten lymph nodes were taken out.

August 15, 2011

Appointment with plastic surgeon at 11:00 a.m.

Second expander inflation. Felt the needle this time—some pain, and a little bleeding. One or two more expansions to go.

August 16, 2011

In a pensive mood today, pondering why I've become overprotective of my kids. Is concern over my condition morphing into unnecessary worry over them? I fret about them driving or riding in a car with friends. James' remark yesterday—"Mom, you are so paranoid"—gave me pause. Why am I so apprehensive about their welfare? Worry sends negative darts. It is like praying for something you don't want!

Remembered something I read: "Unease in the spirit becomes disease in the body."

August 17, 2011

Appointment at medical center at 10:00 a.m.
Electrocardiogram (heart ultrasound)

I've known that "the decision" of whether or not to proceed with chemotherapy was around the corner for weeks now. I've been able to put it out of my mind by concentrating on getting through the surgery.

Now "D" Day (Decision Day) is fast approaching. I have done so much research that my brain is overloaded. I keep coming back to the nagging question: What if I make the wrong decision?

When I was first diagnosed, I was all over the place, searching for that fairy-tale remedy, the solution that would guarantee my cure.

I explored:

- Nutrition
- Juicing
- Herbal supplements
- Acupuncture
- Surgery
- Chemotherapy
- Cancer treatment drugs
- Holistic remedies versus traditional treatments

In hopes of finding "the answer," I've purchased a mountain of books. Marco has been supportive, but expressed that he feels I am grasping at anything anyone recommends. Maybe I am.

I can't believe this is actually happening to me! Sometimes despair just sneaks up on me because of a random thought, something I see on TV, or something I read about.

This morning I was looking at the prescription for my echocardiogram; the doctor had written her reason of concern as "cardio-toxic chemotherapy." Those words jolted me to the core.

The drugs they are recommending can be toxic to the heart, so they want to check the condition of my heart before starting the medications.

Each day is now consumed with the impending decisions regarding what treatments I should accept. But I do feel strongly that the choices are mine to make. It's okay to question protocol. I have to decide based on what I am at peace with for my body!

CHAPTER 9

To Chemo or Not to Chemo?

August 18, 2011

Couldn't sleep. Got up at 4:30 feeling restless. Decided to go for a walk and ended up running—first time post surgery. Felt fabulous to sweat!

Rocked my lopsided boobies in a sports bra and tank top … haha! Tired of "stuffing" to make them look even. Treated myself to some me time in the infrared sauna followed by a sea salt bath. Feel revitalized.

I cringe when I catch a glimpse of my nipple-less, uneven bumps in a mirror. When I touch them, I feel only pressure.

August 19, 2011

I am facing the biggest decision of my life—this outcome cannot be undone.

I am not a scientist or a doctor, but from what I've learned about chemotherapy, I'm not a fan. I'm not sure I want poison circulating through my veins.

Chemotherapy uses chemical agents to kill multiplying cancer cells. Unfortunately, chemo drugs also kill active, growing cells without regard to whether they are cancer cells or noncancer cells.

Chemotherapy treatments are carcinogenic. Many of these drugs list secondary cancers as possible side effects.

Am I leaning against doing chemo because I'm scared of it, or because I'm truly not supposed to put it my body? Could the drugs do more harm than good? I want to weigh all the pros and cons before I make a decision.

Either way, this is scary!

I decided to take out *The Wisdom of Avalon Oracle Cards* (by Colette Baron Reid). I chose these cards from the deck:

> Perception:
> This brings clarity, and asks you to look and wait. Perhaps what you need to do is put on another pair of glasses. Then what is in front of you might be magically transformed. Perception is everything—take no further action until you see how this message applies to your current situation. Then, once you have shifted your perception, you may find that this was all you needed to do.

> Fire Faery:
> The Fire Faery brings creative action and optimism.

> (This Avalon card was oddly mixed in with the Hidden Realms cards.) The Fire Faery signals positive outcomes for your efforts and brings you another gift: illumination.

> When you are in the dark about something, the Fire Faery lends you her light so that your path will be filled with illumination. All things come to light quickly when the Fire Faery appears.

I also pulled these cards from the *Wisdom of the Hidden Realms Oracle Cards* (also by Colette Baron Reid):

Altar Priestess #39:
If all is sacred, how can anything be wrong? Ask how you can shift your consciousness to see your circumstances through the eyes of the Divine, and you will realize how perfect and sacred everything is right now.

Diamond Dreamer #6:
This card speaks of material wealth or true prosperity. The Diamond Dreamer also serves to guide you to the appropriate choices so that the unseen is awakened to move mountains on your behalf. A project finally pays off.

The Lady of Lightning #35:
The Lady of Lightning brings surprises, sometimes shock, and a total paradigm shift. The Lady of Lightning brings powerful forces of change into your life. She tells you to expect a sudden shift in your circumstances. Perhaps a situation you weren't anticipating arises and offers you the opportunity of a lifetime, or a series of "aha" moments culminate in a pivotal flash of insight causing everything to change "just like that." Maybe someone enters your life and pushes you to new heights. You may have a brilliant idea that hits you like lightning.

Be prepared! Change is imminent, and a total paradigm shift may be upon you. Don't resist the changes, as this kind of lightning isn't something you want to fight. Great things are happening when the Lady of Lightning appears!

First post-op appointment with chiropractor Dr. P.

Felt much better afterwards; two weeks of sleeping in a sitting position was not so good for my back.

August 22, 2011

Physical therapy evaluation at 10:00 a.m.

No signs of lymphedema in my arm. No signs of cording (tightening of the tendon). The technician took measurements of my arms, shoulders, and fingers. She gave me information as to what to avoid and signs to look for if I develop future issues with lymphedema.

We went over exercises that stretch the underarm area (which is tight on both sides). She shared that there is a wide range of post-op recovery status with mastectomy patients and that my range of motion is above average. (For some reason that feels like a compliment.)

Came across this quote today (love it!): "To accomplish great things, we must not only act, but also dream; not only plan, but also believe." —Anatole France

August 23, 2011

Appointment for third expansion at 9:15 a.m.

Dr. S said this would most likely be my last expansion; the tissue is healthy enough to accept the implant now. We can schedule the augmentation surgery as soon as we know if I am doing chemo or not.

With each expansion, it gets a bit easier to dress without having to camouflage the size difference. Baby boobie is growing up! I am so ready to get this surgery over with!

I'm feeling anxious about my appointment with the specialist in Miami tomorrow. There is little doubt that he will recommend the Herceptin infusions, but I wonder if he will also recommend chemotherapy.

At a previous appointment with Dr. C, I was astonished to see my oncologist open a website, type in the patient criteria/pathology, and have the software program determine my recommended treatment or "protocol." I have learned to hate that word. I am not comfortable with a computer program (or the organization who devised it) diagnosing me this way. I understand guidelines, but hopefully the doctor has the power to determine the best course of action for the individual patient.

Why do I feel so conflicted? Am I against conventional treatment for the right reasons? I'm starting to question everthing.

Upon learning of my diagnosis almost everyone asks, "How did you find it?" People are always curious about that. I regret that I didn't do self-exams; I could have found it so much earlier.

I was talking with my friend Ali today; she's still having health issues with her legs. She made a point: "Once people know of your affliction, you become defined by it." It is frequently brought up when talking about you, or when inquiring how you have been.

I do not want to be defined by a breast cancer diagnosis; there is so much more to me than that.

I am self-conscious when hugging someone. My breasts feel like coconuts, and I always wonder if the person I'm hugging feels that too.

I've been reading *Women's Bodies, Women's Wisdom: Creating Physical and Emotional Health and Healing* by Christiane Northrup, M.D. Very interesting perspective on how breast cancer can be related to suppression of anger (suppressed immune system), grieving, or unfinished emotional business related to nurturance. She states, "Sometimes the body heals simply when you give yourself permission to listen to its messages."

August 24, 2011

Appointment with oncology specialist in Miami at 1:00 p.m.

I was so happy that Marco was going with me!

As expected, the physician absolutely prescribed Herceptin for the period of one year. He strongly recommended I also do chemotherapy, endorsing the TCH regimen of Taxitear/Carboplatin/Herceptin.

When I relayed that I wasn't keen on the idea of putting toxic chemicals into my body, he said "How about just one? Give it the ole college try. It would make everyone happy." (*Are you kidding me?*)

He continued on, reciting more studies and statistics. After that last comment I heard only, "Blah-blah-blah."

He concurred that it would be okay to have my second surgery first, as they like to start chemotherapy treatment by eight weeks post surgery.

He must have realized that he hadn't persuaded me, because as we were leaving, he advised, "If you are not going to have chemotherapy, at least consider the Herceptin."

Why do physicians downplay the side effects of drugs? Who hasn't seen prescription drug ads on TV showing smiling, active people while a list of debilitating side effects is quietly recited in the background? If a side effect is listed as possible, it has happened to someone.

It was a long, quiet drive home; neither one of us felt like talking. My mind was racing. I just wanted to curl up in a ball and imagine I was watching a movie of someone else's life.

August 25, 2011

When I checked my e-mail this morning I found a Post-it note from Leah on my computer: "Today is a new day!" It made me smile. I need to remember that!

I've been reading *The Healing Code: 6 Minutes to Heal the Source of Your Health, Success, or Relationship Issue* by Alexander Loyd PhD. Dr. Loyd recommends a simple six-minute daily do-it-yourself healing technique to heal the source of any health problem. I'm going to start the routine today!

Distress at the cellular level becomes disease, so you must heal the issue that gave you the stress.

Finally, after a *lot* of soul searching, I have decided not to do any chemotherapy. But I feel I should agree to take the Herceptin infusions. My intention is to supplement conventional treatment with holistic therapies.

I feel at peace with this decision.

August 26, 2011

Appointment with oncologist at 8:30 a.m.

Re-test of pathology showed the same results.

Echocardiogram results were very good: 70.9 percent (anything over 55 percent is good)

When Dr. C asked how my appointment in Miami had gone, I conveyed that the doctor had also advised that I follow the "protocol" of TCH treatments.

As the conversation continued, I needed to let her know I had made up my mind. I started, "Dr. C, I have a lot of respect for you and I am certainly not discounting your expertise, but I have to tell you, I have decided not to do the chemotherapy." She clearly wasn't thrilled with my choice, but seemed somewhat understanding. I found it odd that she asked, "Was he disappointed that he couldn't talk you into it?" (This made me wonder if the "second opinion" was just a "backup" plan to persuade me to follow protocol.)

After confirming that I intended to take the Herceptin infusions, we went on to discuss the benefits. I mentioned my concern about the potential of having a negative effect on the heart.

She reiterated that she wished I would consider chemotherapy because "It has not been recommended to do Herceptin alone. They do not have the data supporting that."

When I asked if she had other HER2+ patients who had done Herceptin without chemotherapy she replied, "Yes. Some have had no recurrence, but others, who had tumors smaller than yours, have had recurrence." She said, "It is a bizarre type, but it can be bizarre in a good way."

She acknowledged that last year my cancer criteria would not have been treated as aggressively as it was this year. Adjuvant treatment was not recommended for anything under a quarter inch.

I'm wondering why that protocol changed.

Knowing that pharmaceutical companies conduct drug trials, I mentioned that the system seems like a conflict of interest and makes me question how accurately the results are obtained and reported.

I left the appointment feeling relief that we can move forward with a treatment plan.

August 30, 2011

Spent some time in quiet reflection this morning. During a self-healing Reiki treatment, I thought about the five Reiki principles and I was reminded that the mind controls the body.

The five Reiki principles:

1. Just for today, I will not be angry. (Letting go of anger brings peace into the mind.)
2. Just for today, I will not worry. (Letting go of worry brings healing into the body.)
3. Just for today, I will be grateful. (Being thankful brings joy into the spirit.)

4. Just for today, I will do my work honestly. (Working honestly brings abundance into the soul.)
5. Just for today, I will be kind to every living thing. (Being kind brings love into the will.)

Appointment with plastic surgeon at 11:00 a.m.

Fourth expansion today – "The Incredible Growing Boobie, Part 4"

Raging rash on my right breast—itchy blisters (maybe she is angry!).

September 7, 2011

It seems as if people I know are looking at me differently now.

Some have remarked (with a surprised tone) about how good I look. So they expect me to look sickly?

Sometimes I feel embarrassed about having breast cancer. Will people think of me as damaged? I always took pride in being healthy.

September 9, 2011

Pre-op appointment with plastic surgeon at 11:00 a.m.

I used to be uninhibited about someone seeing my breasts; now I don't even want to look at them. No more topless parades for these girls!

Dr. S and I discussed expectations for surgery:

- Replace expander with implant
- Replace right implant with larger one

- Remove pockets of fat/tissue below both breasts
- Should take approximately two hours

Dr. S gave his consent for the acupuncturist to be with me during surgery.

When his medical assistant was going over the surgery forms with me, she actually asked, "Do you have nipples?" Well, that's a new one! I've never been asked that question before!

Surgery is scheduled for September 16 at 8:30 a.m. I'm glad we didn't need to postpone the procedure because of this stupid rash.

September 13, 2011

Hospital pre-op appointment at 8:00 a.m.
Acupuncture at 10:00 a.m.

Blood draw—again. Met with the anesthesiologist.

Took an Epsom salt bath and tried one of Alexander Loyd's healing code procedures for the first time—anything is worth a try.

Last "girl maintenance" before surgery—no more shaving allowed until after the procedure. Hope the surgeon doesn't mind hairy armpits!

September 14, 2011

Wanting to get everything in order before my procedure, I did laundry, washed all the bedding, organized the pantry, and tackled anything else I could think of!

I've been reading about an herbal tea that is supposed to have healing benefits. Essiac tea is a product that is composed of four or more herbs, including sheep sorrel and burdock root, which are known to kill cancer cells. Additional herbs help the body detox and build the immune system. A Canadian nurse, Rene Caisse, discovered the formula and, challenging the establishment, successfully treated cancer patients. I wouldn't feel confident using only this regimen, but I certainly believe it could be an effective supplemental remedy.

A news segment regarding cancer on TV today stated that pharmaceutical companies are developing oral chemo drugs for most types of cancer but they are expected to cost about 25 percent more than drugs administered intravenously. They talked about a woman whose cancer had returned; she applied for disability insurance due to having two holes in her hip. She was declined. The insurance company has the discretion to determine who is disabled (due to the ERISA act: The Employee Retirement Income Security Act of 1974). If you choose to go to court and win, there is no additional penalty or fee for the company.

The rash is a lot better; the redness is lighter and the area is smaller. I did a Reiki treatment today and felt better.

September 15, 2011

Surgery tomorrow. I'm not looking forward to going through the whole process again. Just healed from the last one. Ugh! I hate the feeling of my skin being pulled tight. Plus I'm back to limitations in driving, lifting, exercising, reaching.

Not mentally up for another procedure. I just want to be well!

September 16, 2011

We walked into the hospital at 7:30 a.m., and the receptionist told me I was supposed to be there by 7:00 a.m.. How did I get that wrong? I was already nervous, and now I felt awful about being late.

The pre-op nurse who came to get me was very sweet. She told me to forget about the time and not to worry. She said, "We have plenty of time to do what we need to do." Her small act of kindness instantly put me at ease.

We walked through the huge automatic doors that led to the pre-op area, and I found myself entering the same curtained room that I had been in last time. She instructed me to remove all clothing and put the gown on with the opening in the back. Unfortunately, I knew the drill! When the nurse returned, she placed a heated blanket over the bed covers. Of course I had to make a joke about the spa treatment.

Then it was time to start the IV in my hand; I was pleasantly surprised that it didn't hurt at all. She did a great job.

A parade of staff members came by to introduce themselves, including the nurses who would be in the operating room with me, the anesthesiologist, and the assistant anesthesiologist.

The surgical nurse who had been with me during my first surgery peeked around the curtain to say hello and wish me luck. So nice of her! They probably don't have a lot patients come back for seconds.

Dr. N came in to do a pre-op acupuncture treatment. When Dr. D entered the room, I exclaimed, "There is the star"! What? Was I already on medication? How embarrassing!

Dr. S asked if I had any questions, so I told him, "I know we already talked about it, but I was a full C cup before all of this and I would like to get as close to that as possible." He asked me how much bigger—10-20-30 percent? I told him thirty, but after he left, I wondered if that was the right thing to say. I'm not sure how percentage translates into breast size.

The assistant anesthesiologist returned and said, "I'm going to give you something in your IV to relax you." They opened the curtain and started to wheel my bed out, and that is the last thing I remember.

I woke up in recovery in so much pain! The acupuncturist had left the hospital, so I asked for something to relieve the pain. Eventually someone brought me crackers and said I should eat them first. I overheard one of the nurses complaining that they were short staffed. I was moved to a second recovery area and greeted by a nurse who promptly dispensed my medication. I dozed off and felt much better when I awoke, so I asked if I could go home. She replied, "Sure! Whenever you are ready. I was just letting you rest." Marco helped me get dressed, and then he went downstairs to get the car. I was so happy to be heading home.

September 17, 2011

The rash has returned, again! Ugh! Okay, now this rash gets a name; I'll call her Ruby! Itchy red bumps on my breasts, under my breasts, on my chest above my breasts, on my stomach, on my back. Plus, there are welts where the sticky contact pads were!

I summoned the courage to look in the mirror and wished I hadn't. I am very upset! On top of all this, to me, my breasts seem to be the same size they were after the first surgery.

A friend called to see how I was doing and probably wished she hadn't. I vented! I just want to look like I used to! She told me I was beautiful inside and out. I don't feel beautiful, and I feel as if I've lost my sexuality.

Zoe called and offered to come over or take me somewhere to get out for a while. I thanked her but told her I am not up for it. I would not have been good company.

September 19, 2011

Post-op appointment with plastic surgeon at 10:00 a.m.
My pain is very minimal today; only taking an occasional Tylenol.

I told Dr. S that I'm not happy with the size. He recommended we let it heal for a while and see how I feel then. I can tell that he genuinely wants me to be happy with the results.

I started to tear up. Why have I become so emotional? He sweetly handed me a tissue. He probably wanted to get me out of there.

I asked him about the swishing noise I hear in my breasts, and he said it is normal and will go away. He also explained that he had to make small incisions under each breast to remove the excess skin.

I can stop taking the antibiotic; maybe it's the culprit causing the rash?

Follow-up appointment in two weeks.

September 21, 2011

Dr. N (Holistic medicine) was featured on the local news tonight. The segment addressed using integrated medicine for cancer patients.

Dr. H (breast surgeon) also spoke about how he believes alternative therapy can be beneficial for their patients who cannot tolerate pain medication due to adverse reactions. They managed her post surgery pain and recovery with acupuncture treatments.

September 22, 2011

Dermatologist appointment at 8:30 a.m.
Yet another doctor added to the team

I can't believe Ruby is back! I feel like I've been itching for three months now!

- First breakout after biopsy—May 24
- Second after surgery—July 13
- Third mid-August
- Fourth after surgery—September 16

The dermatologist suggested it could be a reaction to the surgery prep solution. She recommended steroid pills and cortisone lotion. I'm reluctant to take steroids because of the negative side effects.

On a happier note, I'm feeling good otherwise with very little discomfort from the surgery.

September 23, 2011

Acupuncture appointment at 4:00 p.m.

It's the weekend, and I should be looking forward to sleeping in tomorrow and having some sexy time with my husband. Instead,

I feel anxiety about that; I don't want to be awkward. I'm self-conscious about the new me.

September 27, 2011

Finally gave in and started taking a prednisone steroid today; I would typically avoid taking a steroid because they can suppress the immune system. But this itchy rash is making me crazy! It heals in one area and then shows up in another. Now it is on my upper chest, neck, and arms.

September 28, 2011

I woke up at 3:00 a.m., probably due to side effect of the prednisone. Since I couldn't go back to sleep, I made the most of my insomnia with some Reiki and meditation.

September 29, 2011

Appointment with oncologist at 9:00 a.m.

We set up the schedule for Herceptin infusions starting on October 7, with additional infusions every three weeks. The medication stays active in your system for six weeks after each infusion. The recommended treatment period is one year.

My understanding of the way Herceptin works is that the antibodies coat the HER2 receptors, which blocks them from communicating with each other. This keeps them from reproducing, and they die.

Dr. C said I could expect to experience flu-like symptoms after the first dose; the initial dose is actually a triple dose. Since subsequent doses are singular, I should tolerate it much better after that.

October 2, 2011

We had a great weekend; our dear friends from Georgia came to visit. It was so much fun to spend time with them and show them around our little town!

October 3, 2011

I've been noticing lately that people are particularly edgy and moody. Is it a full moon? Is Mercury in retrograde?

Interactions with negative people can steal your positive energy and leave a negative void if we allow it. When someone yells at you, offends you, or disrespects you, it's easy to become angry and then take it out on someone else. Energy can be contagious.

I try to pause and remember to be kind because you never know what might be going on in someone's life.

This clearing exercise works great to repel or repair a negative intrusion: Stand with both palms on top of your head. With a sweeping motion from head downwards, extend fingertips and shake hands as if repelling water while straightening arms. Repeat three times while repeating the word *clearing* three times. Visualize positive energy replacing any negative energy.

October 4, 2011

Appointment with plastic surgeon at 2:45 p.m.

The implants have settled in a bit. Circumference is one inch larger. Dr. S said he could increase the implant fluid at the same time as nipple reconstruction if I decide to do it. We're going to wait and see how they look at my next appointment in six weeks.

October 5, 2011

Acupuncture appointment with Dr. N at 9:00 a.m.

Zoe has been curious about acupuncture, so she went with me today.

She snapped a picture of me on the table with an acupuncture needle in between my eyes. Nice souvenir!

Perfect end to a great day—*Survivor* is on tonight! I haven't missed an episode since the first show! I'm looking forward to curling up on the sofa.

October 7, 2011

Morning: Well, the day has arrived—Herceptin Day—my first infusion.

I have to be there at 9 a.m. I'm feeling tense. I hope that my body responds in a positive way. Good-bye, you little bastard cells, *Good-bye!*

Evening:

Shortly after checking in at the reception window, Marco and I were greeted by a friendly nurse who led us back to the "infusion room."

We entered a large area. Looking past the nurses' station, I saw more than twenty recliners lined against the pale walls of the room. A full-size pillow had been placed on every chair, and each space was complete with a side table and portable IV pole. She told me to pick a seat.

As I looked around, it took everything within me not to turn and run out the door. I was overwhelmed. I couldn't believe I was actually standing in a room surrounded by people hooked up to chemo bags. The range in patient ages struck me; it's true that cancer does not discriminate.

I did not want to be there. I was more apprehensive about putting that substance into my body than I had been about having surgery. I was nervous about what side effects I might encounter from taking the medication.

I chose a recliner near the nurses' station, and Marco pulled up a small chair to sit next to me. I looked up at him and immediately had to look away. The empathy in his eyes almost made me fall apart. I felt so many things at that very moment; if one tear had escaped it would have become a river. He whispered something about how brave I am. I do not feel brave. I was so grateful to have him holding my hand.

As the nurse started the IV in my hand, she said, "Let me know if you start itching, and I'll stop the IV immediately." Oh, hell, no! After the Ruby rash, I wasn't taking that chance! I told her that Dr. C had said I would receive Benadryl˚ prior to the Herceptin. She replied that they don't typically pre-medicate with Herceptin but agreed to go check with my oncologist.

She returned and said it had been an oversight. Glad I'd asked!

She handed me two tablets of Tylenol to be taken orally. Benadryl and Zantac would be administered through the IV in addition to Herceptin.

While waiting for my "cocktail," I struck up a conversation with the lady in the recliner next to me. She disclosed that she had gone through a lumpectomy for a six-centimeter tumor, followed by radiation and chemotherapy treatments. She had endured complete hair loss. Having already lost a few fingernails, both of her hands were placed in bowls of ice to hopefully lessen the effects of the regimen on her nails. Noticing that they kept replacing her empty IV bags, I asked her what medications she was taking. Her reply: "I don't know, and I don't want to know." She went on to reveal that she had done absolutely no research. I was surprised when she mentioned that she was a middle school teacher. Here was an educated woman who was so fearful that she didn't want to be informed.

The loading dose of Herceptin is three "servings," each of which takes thirty minutes with a vein flush afterwards. Thankfully, the Benadryl relaxed me within minutes, and I drifted off into a light sleep.

Started Benadryl at 10:00 a.m.
Herceptin at 10:30 a.m.
Finished at 12:15 p.m.

I felt good afterwards with no apparent reaction to the medication. I was just tired, but that was probably due to the Benadryl. Marco and I celebrated by going out to lunch!

I am so relieved I did not have a negative reaction. Thank you, healing angels, for hanging out with me today!

CHAPTER 10
My Body Feels Toxic

October 13, 2011

Chiropractic adjustment at 10:00 a.m.

I've been experiencing some side effects from the Herceptin. The symptoms started a couple of days ago: headaches and sinus drip most of the morning; also some nausea and low back pain

Scheduled a biopsy for the reproductive system issue. I was able to put it out of my mind for a few months, but now Dr. W's office has called twice asking me to schedule. Not exactly looking forward to that!

I watched the television movie *Five* today. It is a collection of short stories about five women who were diagnosed with breast cancer. It touched on how the diagnosis can affect the way women perceive themselves and how it also impacts the lives of the people who love them. Insightful and thought provoking!

October 18, 2011

Yesterday I saw someone wearing a T-shirt that said "Breast Friends." Love it!

Feeling extremely fatigued today. Experiencing strange spasms to right of my belly button and below my breasts in the middle. It's a weird sensation.

October 24, 2011

Had EKG, chest X-ray, and labs today in preparation for biopsy procedure.

I'm not feeling well today, having diarrhea and fatigue.

October 25, 2011

Appointment for lab blood work at 8:45 a.m.

Appointment with Dr. W (gynecologist) 9:50 a.m.

It was my first time back in Dr. W's office since the day she discovered the lump in my breast; little did I know that day, how much my world was going to change.

Today I was so happy to see her. When she came in, I gave her a big hug and thanked her for finding the tumor, for saving my life. She replied that she should be the one hugging me after all I've been through.

I relayed to Dr. W that my breast cancer surgeon had commended her on doing a good job discovering the mass. She smiled saying she was pleasantly surprised at how well I am doing, in such a short period of time.

We discussed the biopsy procedure scheduled for next week. Surgery is at noon; then I should expect an hour and half in recovery.

October 26, 2011

The return of "Ruby the Rash" again! Are you kidding me? I have got to find out what is causing this. Wondering if it is a prep solution used in the operating room.

October 27, 2011

Headache and nausea *all day!*

October 28, 2011

Second Herceptin infusion at 9:00 a.m.

I took an oral Benedryl at home prior to treatment because the IV drip takes an extra thirty minutes. I felt okay afterwards, just tired again. I got this!

Ruby has left the building; thankfully it was a short visit this time!

November 1, 2011

Uterine biopsy with hysteroscopy at 10:45 a.m.

Nurse Mary escorted me from the waiting room back through the double doors to the surgery pre-op area. After stepping onto the scale, I was told to change into the lovely hospital gown; the finishing touch—a stunning blue paper hair cap.

Once I had settled onto the bed, she tried to start the IV. Something went wrong, and the fluid went down into my hand instead of the vein. I am wondering if it is because the same vein was used on

Friday for Herceptin infusion. She said she could have hit a valve; now that didn't sound good! She decided to use the subcutaneous vein inside my elbow instead. I asked her to place the blood pressure cuff on my leg instead of my arm, since I have to use my left arm for all blood work due to lymph node removal on the right side.

The anesthesiologist came in and introduced himself; he was very chatty. I liked him until after he had left and I found out that he had ordered an oral potion for me. The nurse described it as a very bad margarita without the tequila, and crushed up sweet tarts with a lot of salt. Her description was accurate; it tasted terrible! Supposedly it was a stomach antacid. Never drinking that again. Still tasting it at 11:30 p.m.!

The vile potion was followed with some "happy juice" through the IV, and I began to relax. I was feeling lightheaded as they wheeled me into the operating room. Noticing that there wasn't much room to walk around my gurney, I remarked that the room was very small. The nurse retorted with, "It's good enough for what we do here." As I was losing consciousness, I remember hoping I hadn't annoyed her!

While I was in recovery, Dr. W spoke with my husband and explained the process and showed him a digital photo taken during the procedure. I'm quite sure he didn't appreciate that visual!

November 4, 2011

I didn't have to wait for my appointment to find out the results. Dr. W called with the pathology report today; it is benign! Thank you, Universe!

November 8, 2011

Appointment with plastic surgeon at 11:00 a.m.

We discussed adding volume, nipple reconstruction, and nipple tattoos. The assistant showed me photos of other patients' results. The tattoos look so real.

November 10, 2011

Made surgery appointment for December 7. I've decided to add some volume to my implants; hope I am making the right decision. Every time I'm getting dressed, I notice that my bras and tops do not fit. I have a hard time finding something to wear. Dr. S said filling them more should make them a bit rounder—maybe.

November 14, 2011

Appointment with oncologist at 10:00 a.m.

Pulling out my list, I told Dr. C about the symptoms I've been experiencing—sinus drip, shortness of breath, fatigue, and headaches.

Maybe she was running behind, but instead of looking at me when we were speaking, she had her back to me typing on the computer! It was annoying. I think it is rude when a doctor does that.

She responded that the sinus drip was most likely due to smoke in the air from local fires. I disagreed. Then she suggested that my shortness of breath could be due to the implants being heavy on my chest, and this irritated me. They do not feel weighty at all.

I was getting frustrated at not being taken seriously about the symptoms I was experiencing and pointed out that both sinus drip and shortness of breath have been reported as possible side effects of Herceptin.

Addressing my shortness of breath, she recommended that I see a pulmonary specialist; her staff was able to procure an appointment for me next Tuesday. She also sent me to the medical center for a chest X-ray and echocardiogram.

I will see her again in three weeks. When I enquired if I should go ahead with my Herceptin infusion scheduled for Friday, she said it would be fine to delay it until Monday.

I'm concerned that another infusion could exacerbate the symptoms I am already experiencing. I just know I am not feeling right.

November 15, 2011

Appointment with pulmonary specialist at 08:30 a.m.

After a short discussion, he ordered a pulmonary evaluation. It is an outpatient test that will have to be done at the medical center. I'm tired of these doctor appointments taking over my life.

November 16, 2011

Follow-up appointment with Dr. W at 9:00 a.m.

Everything looks great. She reconfirmed that the biopsy was benign. Check that off the list.

Pulmonary respiratory test at 2:30 p.m.

The test consisted of a series of breathing exercises; it took about an hour. When we were halfway through, the technician had me exhale completely and then draw deeply from an inhaler with medication that dilated the airway. I felt like I was on speed! We should have the results sometime next week.

November 17, 2011

Called Dr. H's office to find out whether or not there had been cancer cells on the chest muscle. I remembered reading on a report that the cells were suspected, I also recalled someone telling me they were not present. I just want to know for sure.

Dr. H personally returned my call this evening and explained that the MRI in June showed suspicion of cells on the pectorals muscle. So he had taken some of the muscle tissue for testing, and pathology had confirmed it was free of carcinoma. Genuinely invested, he asked me how I was doing and enquired about my present treatment.

I asked what I should do for follow-up screening; I know I will no longer require mammograms, but what about ultrasounds? He said the oncologist will do follow up exams and order any diagnostics if necessary. Then he added, "But I'm always here if you have a concern or question." What a great doctor!

November 20, 2011

Herceptin Infusion #3 at 9:30 a.m.

It took three tries for them to get a vein—uggh! Again the same problem with the vein in my hand—it blew. It was painful, and my hand hurt for hours afterward. Finished the treatment around 11:30 a.m. It looks like even my veins are no longer willing participants.

I didn't take Benadryl this time; it makes me sleepy.

November 21, 2011

Appointment with pulmonary specialist at 11:15 a.m.

The pulmonary test had indicated a decreased function in my airways, most likely caused by the Herceptin, as respiratory issues are a possible side effect.

But while dictating his report into a recorder, I heard him say "Pulmonary respiratory disease." Interrupting him, I questioned, "Now I'm labeled as having respiratory disease?" He paused for a moment and reworded his report explaining it was decreased pulmonary function caused by pharmaceutical treatment. He determined that medication was not necessary to treat the shortness of breath since it wasn't impeding my daily activities.

I realized how easily information could be misconstrued and become a part of my permanent record.

December 2, 2011

At my acupuncture today, we discussed the respiratory issues I have been experiencing. He focused treatment on the lung meridian points; at the end of the session, my breath capacity was improved.

December 7, 2011

Reconstruction surgery number three with Dr. S
Surgery center at 9:30 a.m. Home by noon.

How does that phrase go? Third time's the charm?

The incisions are minimal. I have slight discomfort on the right side, but not bad enough for pain meds. The implants definitely look bigger.

December 9, 2011

Appointment with the oncologist at 8:00 a.m.

I vocalized my concerns about the decreased pulmonary function. Dr. C assured me that she is very cautious about damage caused by medications and would stop the Herceptin if started to cause issues.

She is going to submit an official scientific question to the cancer society to enquire if any lung toxicity issues have been reported.

We discussed my cancer markers; they are all normal. That's definitely good news! Will continue to check markers every six weeks.

December 10, 2011

"Ruby the Rash" is back. OMG...again? My breasts look huge, and the skin is stretched so tight; what have I done? I hope it is just due to the swelling. My worst fear was going too big. Hope I didn't make a mistake.

December 12, 2011

Herceptin infusion at noon

The infusion went fine, but afterwards I asked the nurse to see if Dr. C would give me a prescription for prednisone for the rash. She came back and said that they would need to see me first to make sure it wasn't an infection. I was sent back to the waiting room.

An hour passed before I was called back to an examination room. Shortly after, the assistant returned to escort me back to the waiting room. She explained that the wait would be shorter for the nurse practitioner and a room would be opening soon.

Forty-five minutes later, I found myself in another examination room listening to the nurse practitioner telling me that she would need the doctor to come take a look.

When I think of the number of appointments, tests, treatments, and surgeries I've endured since my diagnosis, it seems as if I've lived in the reception and exam rooms of countless doctors. I don't even want to know how many hours I've spent doing this.

Finally I walked out the door with my prescription in hand, but no one can tell me what keeps causing this allergic reaction.

Deep breath...tomorrow is another day.

December 13, 2011

Woke up this morning with a runny nose, sore throat, and cough. Started the methylprednisolone pack today for this damn rash. Surprised I am still losing weight.

December 16, 2011

Side effects from the Herceptin infusion are more intense this time. They include decreased pulmonary function, shallow breathing, nasal drip, cough, sore throat, nasty medicine taste in my mouth, plus a lack of taste when I eat. I'm seriously thinking about telling Dr. C I don't want to continue the infusions. I'm concerned about the potential of irreversible respiratory damage.

December 19, 2011

Post-op appointment with Dr. D at noon

I'm healing well, but they feel huge! Maybe it's just that I had gotten accustomed to having smaller breasts. It has been five months since my mastectomy.

December 25, 2011

Christmas at our house! We had twenty people for dinner; I was so happy to be hosting the holiday! We exchanged gifts, played games, and enjoyed the delicious food. The "*C*" word didn't cross my mind, not even once.

December 29, 2011

Oncologist appointment with Dr. C at 08:00 a.m.

I'm still having breathing issues and have developed a persistent cough. These are asthma-type symptoms.

I told Dr. C that I want to stop the Herceptin infusions. Unless it is very shallow, every time I take a breath I have to cough. It is has been happening daily for almost three weeks now. We discussed that the pulmonary specialist had concluded that the respiratory issues were related to the Herceptin medication.

Dr. C is going to speak with one of the developers of Herceptin about my symptoms/reaction.

I just know my body doesn't feel right. I'm extremely fatigued. I'm not sure I will be keeping the appointment for my next Herceptin infusion.

December 31, 2011

It's New Years Eve! I am sooo ready to say good-bye to 2011!

January 2, 2012

I feel like the Herceptin is at a toxic level in my body. I can taste the medicine after my infusions, and I smell it when I go to the bathroom. I'm thinking I should skip the next dose, which is scheduled for the day after tomorrow. It seriously feels as if I'm developing asthma.

January 4, 2012

I called and left a message with my oncologist's office, just waiting for her reply regarding my desire to discontinue the infusions. It has been twelve weeks of treatment now.

Someone recently mentioned to me that there is a clinical trial, taking place in Europe, in which participants are taking Herceptin without adjunct chemotherapy, and the duration of treatment is actually twelve weeks-not twelve months. Interesting. Why is this course of treatment being considered in Europe but not in the United States?

January 9, 2012

I feel sick to my stomach and fatigued. I still have a cough, diarrhea, and feel congested. Not a great day.

January 10, 2012

Appointment with plastic surgeon at 10:00 a.m.

Maybe I am just being unreasonable? The size feels too big, especially at the top, seems like they start at my collarbone. I thought I wanted them bigger, but now I am self-conscious. It feels like something is poking me in the left breast, and I cannot move the breast as I can the right one.

Dr. S listened then suggested I give it a couple months, adding that we have options. We could remove some fluid or exchange the implant to a teardrop shape. It takes time for the implants to settle.

January 12, 2012

Appointment with oncologist at 4:30 p.m.

Dr. C relayed that she had spoken with the pulmonary specialist, and he had found no signs of toxicity in lungs, just airway reactivity. Isn't the airway reaction due to toxicity? She then inserted that I would be a rare case, as she wasn't aware of previous reports of pulmonary toxicity caused by this medication. First report—lucky me!

I showed her the printout of information I found on a legitimate website stating that pulmonary toxicity is rare (less than 1 percent) and usually happens shortly after the first dose (first dose is triple) but can occur with second or later doses.

She reminded me that my family history states my mother had asthma. I said, "I have never had a hint of respiratory issues prior to now; that would be quite a coincidence."

She went on to say that maybe I could be having a reaction to the globin in the medication and suggested we try a lower dose—one-third once a week instead of a full dose once every three weeks. I'm still in limbo as to whether or not to even continue infusions; I wasn't sure I was on board with that solution. Since she doesn't support stopping the medication, I don't feel comfortable making that call; I was hoping for a little more confirmation before making that choice.

She acknowledged, "We don't know if you haven't had enough," but then she re-iterated that the recommended dosage is every three weeks over a one year period.

She reminded me that, statistically, my possibility of reoccurrence is at least 35 percent without chemotherapy and Herceptin. I could regret not completing the twelve-month regimen.

We agreed to also skip the next treatment (January 25) and meet with her in three weeks. Hopefully by then I can confirm whether or not to continue the infusions.

January 13, 2012

Went for a run today. It felt awesome! But soon after I got home, my breath became shallow and I started coughing. This sucks!

January 24, 2012

I have skipped two infusions. It's been about six weeks, and I'm definitely feeling better, breathing more deeply, and the cough has dissipated considerably.

The possible recurrence rate was concerning, but I had to weigh my present quality of life against a statistic that might not have applied to my case. I'm actually more troubled by the possibility of permanent damage to my pulmonary system if I continue the medication.

February 6, 2012

Appointment with oncologist at 4:00 p.m.

When Dr. C entered the exam room and asked how I was feeling, I told her I was feeling really good. Pulmonary symptoms have subsided almost completely, and my energy level is much better.

Her response, in a slightly surprised tone, was, "So you did have toxicity." What, now you believe me?

"I have talked to a million people about you," she said. "I found one doctor who had one patient who had pulmonary toxicity." When I asked, "What did that patient do"? she replied that the patient had stopped the medication. I wanted to know how long the patient had been taking it, but she said she hadn't asked.

Thinking out loud, Dr. C was trying to find a solution. "You could try taking the pill form of Herceptin. The side effects include acne and diarrhea." (Now that sounds like fun!) Then she interjected that we would have to ask the doctor in Miami if he thinks I should switch to the pill method. That approach has never been used for a case like mine; it has been used only for cancers that have metastasized.

As our conversation came to an end, we agreed that I would stop the medication and restart the infusions at a later time if needed.

She wants to monitor me closely and see me more often than she typically sees other patients, and she recommended that I go for a CAT scan every six months.

Expressing that I would rather not do CAT scans if they are not completely necessary; I voiced concern about radiation exposure. She understood and agreed that we could monitor blood markers, which is one of the first and most accurate indicators.

I am comfortable with discontinuing the medication because my margins were clear, no lymph nodes were involved, and the cut-off for recommending chemo is 2.0 centimeters. My tumor measured 2.2 centimeters.

Dr. C mentioned that I wouldn't have qualified for the initial US study of Herceptin because my prognosis wasn't bad enough since mine was lymph node negative. I am so grateful to the ladies who were brave enough to do that trial. Even though I had a reaction, I still believe Herceptin was instrumental in my healing and the destruction of my cancer cells.

Although, having said that, I am conflicted about the fact that US drug trials are run by pharmaceutical companies. Why would they recommend shorter terms for treatment when they can extend their financial income? Cancer is big business; why "remedy" something that built one of the largest profitable industries?

With the massive fundraising for breast cancer research, I wonder how much is actually spent on finding a cure. Are any of these funds put toward discovering alternative solutions, or are they used solely to develop and market poisonous substances?

Isn't it possible that the answer could lie within less-toxic methods?

I am so glad that I questioned the necessity of chemotherapy in my case, and happy that I listened to my body when toxicity was raising its ugly head.

I realize that chemo may be necessary in some situations, but all too often, it is served up as a precaution. Many people do not realize that chemo can and does cause residual cancers.

CHAPTER 11

My New Normal

February 17, 2012

Today I started Dr. Andrew Weil's life-balancing breathing exercises.

Twice a day, morning and evening, I practice Dr. Weil's breathing meditation, which goes like this:

1. Take a deep breath in through mouth and release it through nose.
2. Breathe in through nose to the count of four.
3. Hold that breath to the count of seven.
4. Release the breath through the mouth to the count of eight, with force and sound.

I repeat this four times, and then I visualize being at my favorite beach spot, and I clear my thoughts.

February 21, 2012

Appointment with plastic surgeon at 3:30 p.m.

We discussed a procedure to remove some of the saline and relieve some pressure. I feel as if there are two coconuts sitting on my chest. Also, the port is poking me in the left breast. Will this party ever end?

February 23, 2012

Appointment with massage therapist at 10:00 a.m.

My right arm feels fatigued, achy, and a bit swollen. I went for a lymphatic drainage treatment; she also treated the incision area with a machine that is supposed to decrease and soften scar tissue.

March 9, 2012

Surgery number four today to reduce size at 2:30 p.m.

Hoping to eliminate the shelf effect at top of breasts and bulging at sides by armpits. Dr. S changed the surgery prep solution, and I still developed a rash after surgery. Could it be the antibiotic?

Another round of prednisone; I hate compromising my immune system by putting that into my body. This time I had more pain upon awakening than last time—a burning and stinging pain in both breasts. I am so done with this routine.

March 26, 2012

The implants felt better on my post-op appointment eleven days ago. Not so full and tight. The results from my last blood draw came in today. Everything looks good, within normal range, and my marker numbers are great! Scheduled my next appointment in three months; I have graduated to a longer stretch between marker checks. *Yay!*

March 29, 2012

Post-op appointment with plastic surgeon at 8:45 a.m.

It has been three weeks since surgery. The port on the left implant is poking me, and the center area is numb. Also, I feel something in the upper left armpit. These areas are uncomfortable to the touch.

Dr. S said this should subside when the skin stretches more. It is a strange sensation to have foreign objects poking you from the inside.

June 4, 2012

Appointment with medical massage therapist at 4:00 p.m.

During my appointment today the therapist was working around the breast area to soften the fascia and perimeter tissue, as well as check the lymphatic flow.

Maybe it was the realization that I didn't have a sexual response and I just felt pressure against the skin, but I suddenly became emotional, and silent tears spilled over, running down my face.

I was so embarrassed by the display of emotion, but the therapist didn't miss a beat. He was so sweet and assured me that we would work through this process together.

July 13, 2012

The bi-lateral mastectomy surgery to remove the cancer was one year ago today.

I certainly did not know what was ahead of me; all the decisions, uncertainty, and countless hours spent with doctors.

I am not complaining. I am so thankful for where I stand in this cancer craziness. I could have had a very different outcome.

July 16, 2012

Three-month follow up appointment with oncologist at 9:00 a.m.

I've actually been able to put the thoughts of cancer out of my mind over the past few months. But this morning, as I walked into that building, the memories, feelings, and fears came rushing right back. Something inside me tensed as I opened that office door. Pretty sure I will always brace myself when entering there.

After I checked in, I found a seat and waited for my name to be called. As I glanced around the room, again I was reminded that cancer does not discriminate. I saw women and men—young and old, wealthy and not so wealthy, from all walks of life. Many women had their heads covered with wraps or scarves. Some had brought coolers of ice to immerse their nails into during their treatments. I couldn't help but feel sorry for those who looked pale and feeble. Loved ones were accompanying those new to this club. One mother and daughter caught my attention; the mother was having her first chemo treatment, and the daughter's face said it all—she was afraid of losing her mom. The love between them wasn't spoken, but it was too obvious to miss. Then there was the couple who started to argue, quietly at first, but it escalated to the point that forced him to get up out of his seat and spout that he was leaving. He coldly told her to call when she needed a ride home. The entire waiting room went silent; it was awkward, and everyone felt sad. I wanted to go give her a hug. After a few minutes, he returned and quietly told her that he was sorry. This isn't just hard for those who have cancer; it is painful for the people who love them.

I heard my name being called, and I followed the nurse back to the lab room for my blood draw—the dreaded marker check! After my vitals and labs were taken, I was led to the exam room, instructed to remove my top and bra (Bra? Who needs a bra?), and put on the lovely paper vest.

The nurse practitioner came in to review my previous results and said, "Your markers are good ... very good. The numbers are those of someone who has never had cancer."

It took a moment for the words sink in; it was the best news I have had in a very long time! I told her that I actually feel better now than before I was diagnosed.

My next appointment for follow-up will be in six months. A six-month reprieve!

I walked out of that office with a much lighter step than I'd had when I walked in. But I do know that next January, when I return and step back through those doors, I will face the same trepidation I felt today.

July 27, 2012

It's been a long year since that restoring walk on the beach—my first outing after surgery. Of course we had to go back today! It is exactly one year later. I feel healthy from head to toe and, oh, so blessed!

August 15, 2012

James leaves for college tomorrow. We are proud and excited for him, but also a little melancholy. Will he be happy? Will he make good decisions? We are going to miss him so much!

It feels strange knowing this is the last night I will go to bed, close my eyes, and know that he is sleeping nearby in his room … the last night I will know his friends inside out, his mood, if he ate lunch … the last time I know I will see his teenaged sleepy face come downstairs in the morning. Of course he will be home again, but things will be different. He will be an adult.

August 16, 2012

Helped James move into his dorm room today. Thus begins the next chapter in his life.

August 29, 2012

Took a yoga and meditation class this morning. Just what I needed— some me time!

One of my favorite affirmations:

"I invite the power of love, light, and transformation."

September 04, 2012

I thought I was doing just fine adjusting to James being away at college. Maybe it's bothering me more than I thought.

After years of constantly looking after his every need, I feel as if I am in a void. I miss him! While they are growing up, you feel that practically every decision is filled with thoughts of your kids. You are crazy busy with appointments, car pools, sleepovers, sports, and proms. It feels as if I just got fired from a job after eighteen years with the company. Knowing that Leah will also be leaving in less than a year doesn't help!

September 19, 2012

Can't believe I'm actually thinking about making an appointment to talk with my plastic surgeon about a revision. Since I've resumed lifting weights at the gym, I've noticed changes in my chest. Maybe it is due to building up the muscle, but there is a constant tightness, and my breasts are sore when I wake up in the morning. I am constantly aware of them and reminded of the foreign objects inside of me.

I wanted to re-create what they were before the mastectomy; but without any breast tissue, that may be unrealistic.

My posture is not good; I find myself slouching to overcompensate. Maybe I need them to be smaller. Maybe I should just totally remove both of them. I can't believe I am sitting here seriously considering another surgery. I'm actually embarrassed to call Dr. S, but this is my body; I am the one who lives here.

September 21, 2012

Sometimes a sudden wave of sadness sneaks up on me. Maybe I'm mourning the loss of my breasts; I miss my nipples. I don't like the sensation of pressure I feel when I lean against something, like when I workout at the gym. When I hug someone, do they feel the implants?

October 21, 2012

I want to feel like a woman again. Tonight I tried to explain to Marco what I've been feeling, and only tears came out. He wrapped his arms around me and told me that they look great … that I look great. That was a most genuine compliment, and he had no idea how much I needed to be reassured of his love at that moment.

January 21, 2013

Appointment with Dr. C at 9:00 a.m.

Sitting there in the parking lot of the oncologist office, I had trepidation in my stomach and fear on my shoulders; that six months of amnesty passed too quickly! I took a deep breath when I walked into that waiting room!

Lab results show that the cancer markers look good. But my B12 level is very low. Going to start weekly injections to raise levels.

Next appointment is in three months, so much for graduating to six months!

January 29, 2013

Appointment with plastic surgeon at 10:00 a.m.

I've been having pain in the left breast; it is very sensitive to the touch, and I can feel the port. Even shower water pressure causes discomfort. Is it possible that I've developed scar tissue or capsular contraction in my left breast?

We discussed switching implants to a smaller size since surgery is necessary anyway.

March 15, 2013

Had my fourth B12 injection today. The doctor determined that the memory and concentration issues I've been experiencing are most likely due to having low B12 levels. It freaked me out to learn how serious an untreated B12 deficiency could be. That vitamin is crucial to so many vital functions in the body. Since my levels are still low, we are going to continue the B12 injections.

I wonder why my B12 levels plummeted. I did not have this issue prior to my cancer diagnosis. Was it a side effect caused by taking the steroids for the revisiting Ruby?

July 13, 2013

Two years cancer free! Woo-hoo!

August 20, 2013

Pre-op appointment with plastic surgeon at 11:00 a.m.

When Dr. S walked in, I was reading a magazine about the victims of the Boston Marathon bombing. I told him that I feel guilty making a fuss about my breasts when they had lost limbs and life. He told me that I shouldn't feel that way, that I too had lost parts of my body I hadn't foreseen losing. Moments like that make him more than just a doctor; they make him a compassionate human being.

August 21, 2013

Appointment at oncologist office for a blood draw. Am I going to have any blood left?

Why are the doors that lead to the exam and treatment rooms always locked? You have to be buzzed in by the receptionist. Who would want to go back there if he or she didn't have to? (I realize it is because of the drugs they store, but it did strike me as funny.)

August 22, 2013

Tomorrow is Leah's turn to leave for college. Feeling the same nostalgia I felt on James' last night home before he left. I tiptoed into her room just to see her sleeping in her bed, just as I did when she was little.

August 23, 2013

We helped Leah move into her dorm room today. My baby girl has moved out, and I am sad that things will never be the same. With both of the kids gone, the house will be so quiet and so empty. I miss my babies! And their noisy friends!

August 27, 2013

Having yet another surgery tomorrow—exchanging the implants and removing scar tissue.

As much as I dread going through this whole procedure and recovery process again, I am now looking forward to downsizing, to not having the discomfort, and to constant awareness that there is a foreign object in my body.

August 28, 2013

Surgery number five, procedure at 10:30 a.m.

Leaving for the surgery center in a few minutes. This is the very last time I am putting my body through this process.

August 31, 2013

The procedure went well and the implants definitely feel better already.

True to form, Ruby the infamous rash has arrived (red, itchy, inflamed blisters)! We have eliminated everything we could think of!

Maybe it's my body reacting to the solution used to clean the pocket and implant prior to insertion. I just hope it isn't a response to the actual implants!

September 1, 2013

Woke up at 2:00 a.m. unable to get comfortable; it feels as if my chest is being pricked with fiery hot needles. Each outbreak of this post-surgery rash is worse than the time before. I have resorted to another round of prednisone. I surrender!

September 3, 2013

Appointment with Dr. C at 8:00 a.m.

The oncologist said that my marker numbers look great; those words always sound like a gift from heaven!

September 20,2013

The augmentation went well. I have full range of motion without discomfort and "Ruby has left the building"! For good!

I've come to the realization that I need to stop trying to replicate my breasts as they were prior to my diagnosis. It is difficult to duplicate the size and shape without any breast tissue, but I'm healing fast and the incisions are barely noticeable anymore.

I realize losing a breast or a nipple doesn't compare to losing a loved one; but somehow the five stages of grief or loss seem to apply. I experienced denial, anger, bargaining, depression, and finally acceptance.

I've come to terms with my new normal. I choose to focus on the fact that I am here and healthy. I am grateful!

CHAPTER 12

Some Moments Change Us

I never dreamed I'd be sitting in a doctor's office hearing the words *you have cancer*. Yet there I was. The diagnosis belonged to me, not a friend, a neighbor, or some stranger. My very own body was betraying me. The impact of those words stunned me. My brain exploded and went numb in the same moment. It was hard to focus, and I couldn't feel my body. Waiting for the biopsy results had been torture. Now the dreaded outcome was indeed my reality.

I've often wondered, why did this become part of my journey? What is the purpose in it? What am I supposed to learn from this situation?

After being diagnosed, I focused on gathering information; I researched everything I could think of relating to breast cancer. I purchased and devoured enough books to start a library, bought any magazine that had the word *cancer* on the cover, and collected every brochure and pamphlet in my path. I was determined to learn everything I could about this beast and to find out how I could beat it. I became obsessed with finding out what caused me to get cancer. Was it something I was eating? Something I was exposed to? Was it that root canal I had done?

Issues in the teeth can block energy flow in acupuncture meridians, and those blockages can weaken corresponding organs and tissues. Some biological (holistic) dentists believe there is a link between root canals and disease in the body. Harmful bacteria thrive in a root canal, and the toxins can travel throughout the body and negatively impact a delicate immune system. A dead tooth is a dead body part. Why would we think it is a good idea to keep it in our mouth?

There are countless causes of cancer, including genetics, environmental exposures, and toxins. Is it also possible that breast cancer can stem from a lack of self-love and nurturing oneself? Maybe. But if our thoughts and feelings can contribute to manifesting illness and disease, couldn't they also help us to manifest healing? I think so! Even the most conventional doctors will tell you that your state of mind can affect your physical health.

Throughout my tug-of-war with cancer, I tried to maintain a positive outlook. I had to come to grips with the unfolding nightmare. Of course I was scared, but I knew that fear is paralyzing, and I wanted to be fearless not fearful!

I understand that the conventional approach may be the best path in some cases, but something in my soul urged me to look at all options before making any decision regarding treatment. Being holistically minded, I wanted alternatives to pumping poison through my veins, being cooked from the inside out, and consuming medications that can actually cause cancer.

Hoping to avoid fear-based decisions and before making vital, life-changing choices, I needed to arm myself with knowledge. Toxic chemotherapy can be more detrimental than cancer itself. I needed to determine if the potential benefits were worth the risks.

Seeking an approach that would nurture and preserve my body, mind, and spirit, I was willing to consider unconventional therapies. Scientifically minded people may be uncomfortable with phenomena they cannot document or understand. Western modalities tend to treat symptoms with pharmaceuticals where Eastern philosophies embrace more natural remedies.

Even though fear of being wrong lingered in the back of my mind, after weeks of soul searching and endless research, I chose to reject chemotherapy treatment. Convinced my best course of action was to balance traditional, alternative, and preventive therapies, I embarked on a path of integrative medicine, which combines modern Western medicine with alternative methods from other parts of the world. This approach encompasses the biological, psychological, and spiritual aspects of health. In addition to addressing my immediate health problem, I wanted to focus on illness prevention and develop healthy habits.

Here is a breakdown of some of the treatments and therapies I utilized.

Conventional treatments:

- Surgery: bi-Lateral mastectomy with augmentation
- Herceptin infusions

Alternative holistic and preventive treatments:

Acupuncture
This is a form of Chinese medicine that boosts immunity, relieves pain, and alleviates stress.

Vitamins
- Vitamin D3 helps to regulate the expression of genes that influence the immune system and boost the body's ability to fight illness.
- Vitamin B12 affects the development of red blood cells, which is important to the nervous system and adrenal function. It also boosts energy level and supports digestion.

Since I was consumed with fatigue, my doctor ordered a blood test. It was confirmed that my B12 level was very low. I learned that medications I had taken can interfere with B12 levels including the antibiotics sulfamethoxazole and trimethoprim, the prednisone treatment methylprednisolone, and ibuprofen.

Probiotics

Probiotics counter the effects of antibiotics taken during and after surgery.

Essential oils

Essential oils are produced by plants. To extract the oil the plant material is steam distilled. The therapeutic oils contain powerful properties:

- Frankincense is used for immunity and emotional issues. It strengthens the immune system, reduces inflammation, and fades scars.
- Lemon alkalizes the body, cleanses the lymphatic system, and eases fatigue and anxiety.
- Lavender is calming. It relaxes emotions and induces sleep.
- Peppermint is good for the digestive system. It soothes headache, eases nausea, relieves muscle pain, and enhances respiratory health.
- Juvaflex is good for detoxification. It has supportive effects on the liver as well as on the digestive and lymphatic systems.

Therapeutic massage

This provides relaxation, relieves stress, and increases circulation. It can also strengthen the immune system by accelerating the activity level of the body's natural "killer cells" that work to destroy cancer cells.

Infra-red sauna

This expels toxins in the body, stimulates blood circulation, helps to evacuate edema, decreases inflammation, and speeds healing. (A nice side effect is that up to 600 calories are burned in a thirty-minute session!)

Intuitive Pranic healing

This therapy treats the energy body, which in turn treats the physical body. The therapy uses the aura, chakras, and *ki* (Prana, or source of energy) for balancing energy. The seven chakras and their locations are:

- Root: at base of spine
- Spleen or abdomen: below the navel, lower abdomen
- Solar plexus: above the naval, stomach area
- Heart: center of chest
- Throat: throat region
- Third eye: forehead, between the brows
- Crown: top of head

Reiki therapy

This ancient Oriental method of healing uses healing symbols and the universal life force, which balances the flow of energy by releasing blockages.

Illness can be triggered by energy disruption and chakra imbalance in the body. The balance and flow of our energy is vital to our well-being. It underlies the condition—both physical and mental—of our physical bodies.

Exercise and yoga

Physical activity increases oxygen levels and arouses the immune system. Regular exercise boosts energy and also improves mood and quality of sleep.

Yoga builds muscle strength, corrects posture, and increases blood flow. Yoga can stimulate drainage of lymph, the fluid that circulates throughout the lymphatic system. It helps the lymphatic system fight infection, destroy cancerous cells, and dispose of toxic waste products. Yoga can also decrease blood sugar by lowering cortisol and adrenaline levels.

Meditation

Meditation is a mindfulness practice that affects awareness and allows you to filter out mental chatter. Even just a few minutes each day cleanses and nourishes you from within, reducing stress and improving immunity. Dive inside yourself.

"The greatest weapon against stress is our ability to choose one thought over another." —William James

Visualization

Visualization is the technique of creating images by using your imagination to reach goals and generate success. The key to manifesting what you want may lie in your ability to visualize it.

Juicing

Juicing extracts the juice from fruits and vegetables so your body can more effectively absorb the nutrients, which boosts your immune system and aids in removing toxins from your body.

Lemon water every morning prior to breakfast

Drink one large glass of room-temperature water to which you have added the juice of half a lemon or the equivalent (one and a half tablespoons) of bottled organic lemon juice. Lemon juice is a natural diuretic that flushes out toxins. It boosts your immune system, hydrates the lymph system, detoxes the liver, aids in digestion, and balances the body's PH level, reducing overall acidity creating an alkaline environment. Stress produces acid in the body, which creates a friendly environment for cancer to propagate.

Avoiding refined sugar

Sugar is toxic to the body; it feeds cancer, as the rogue cells thrive on it. Consider that the PET scan (positive emission tomography) uses radioactively labeled glucose to detect sugar-hungry tumor cells.

Avoiding processed food and preservatives

Nutrients in food directly impact the mechanisms by which cancer cells grow and spread. They can also indirectly impact cancer by changing the surrounding biochemical conditions that either promote or inhibit the progression of malignant diseases.

Eating organic vegetables and fruit

Include kale, broccoli, lemons, all berries, apples, grapefruit, pomegranate, and watermelon in your diet.

The numbers on organic fruit labels always begin with the number nine and contain five digits. The numbers on genetically modified fruit labels begin with the number eight and often contain five digits. Conventional fruit labels begin with the number four.

Crucial to healing and prevention is eliminating things that are toxic and fuel the growth of cancer. Maintaining an alkaline environment, getting regular exercise, and practicing stress relief are key elements in restoring the body's immune system.

There is a lot of conflicting information out there. Be your own advocate, ask questions, and educate yourself. Get copies of all your lab results so you can compare them; learn what the abbreviations stand for and why the test was ordered. Know about potential side effects of medications. Acquire knowledge so you can proceed subjectively. Cancer is complex, and every diagnosis is unique; pathology results vary with each individual.

I am eternally grateful for the brave women who participated in the Herceptin trials. Knowing that Herceptin targets the specific cells of HER2+ cancer was instrumental in my decision to decline chemotherapy. I have no doubt that the Herceptin infusions played a major role in my healing. But I am also glad I listened to my body and discontinued the treatment when it started to cause toxicity.

Health care is more that just medicine. Many Western-minded physicians do not consider the possibilities and benefits of Eastern treatments. People are uncomfortable with things they do not understand, and especially things that cannot be scientifically explained. Yet there is growing support in the use of holistic modalities. Complementary therapies are more commonly used adjunctive to mainstream care; there is mounting evidence that they can be powerful tools in facilitating healing.

Not doing chemo was the right choice for me in my situation. However, we all have to make our own decisions. It is neither my place nor my intention to tell anyone what lifestyle or treatment choices to make. My message is simply this: empower yourself and be the boss of your body.

I can't say that I follow a particularly strict diet or obsess about my environment. I am mindful, I try to make healthy choices, and I'm conscious of what I put in and onto my body, from food and water to lotions and toothpaste. The most significant change I made was to renounce my sugar habit. It is no secret that refined sugar is toxic to the body, and cancer thrives on it. I also do my best to keep my body at an alkaline PH level. Cancer cells flourish in an acidic system; it's tougher for them to endure an alkaline environment. In order to triumph over cancer, we need to eliminate things that fuel the growth of cancer cells. We all have cancer cells in our bodies. It's important to keep our bodies' defense systems strong in order to defeat defective cells so they don't have a chance to arrange a tumor party!

Everyone knows that stress is harmful to our health. When I feel stressed or need to clear mental clutter, I meditate. It regenerates the mind and soul. Meditation doesn't have to be complicated. You can meditate while taking a walk or a run. Sometimes I simply sit still and pay attention to my breath, allowing thoughts to pass through my consciousness and float away.

Here is one of my favorite healing meditations:

Healing River Journey Meditation
By Eddie Mullins, intuitive counselor

1. Take three deep cleansing breaths.
2. Imagine you are standing on a riverbank.
3. You see a canoe coming toward you with healing angel Isis in it.

4. The canoe stops in front of you and you get in. You bring along anyone you want—Archangel Michael, Archangel Raphael, guides … anyone.
5. As you proceed along the river in the canoe, notice the sky, sun, trees, the breeze. Notice how it all feels.
6. You approach a waterfall. Go through it.
7. The river levels lower as you come out other side of waterfall.
8. The scene is completely new; imagine your peaceful place (beach or mountains or whatever).
9. Get out of the canoe and proceed along the path.
10. Notice what you see along the way-visions, animal totems, guides?
11. You sit down on a large crystal stone.
12. Go into the energy of your pain or source of discomfort and ask what the energy is telling you.
13. What needs to release? What is the message?
14. If thoughts intrude or your mind wanders, bring back focus with breath. Take in all you sense; see and feel everything.
15. When you are ready, proceed back down the path you came on and return to the canoe.
16. When the river levels up, go back under the waterfall.
17. Continue back up the river to the bank, and exit the canoe.
18. Thank those you took on your journey with you.
19. Open your eyes and refresh.

This is an effective breathing practice that is easy to do:

Life Balancing Breathing Exercise
By Andrew Weil, M.D., holistic physician

1. Take a deep breath in through mouth and release it through nose.
2. Breathe in through nose to the count of four.
3. Hold that breath to the count of seven.
4. Release the breath through the mouth to the count of eight, with force and sound. (The force of sound helps to fully empty the lungs.)

Do four breath cycles twice every day.

Benefits:
- Changes the balance in involuntary nervous system
- Lowers blood pressure
- Slows the heart rate
- Improves digestion

We tend to focus on how we look on the outside, but we need to work on taking care of the inside as well. It is important to nurture the mind, body, and spirit.

I wouldn't define myself as a religious person, but I am definitely spiritual. I believe in a higher power. I believe that our spirits live on and that we are here in human vehicles to better our souls. We are on this earthly realm to overcome challenges and negativity. We have the ability to set things in motion.

There are countless angels available to assist us; my two favorites are Archangel Raphael, who facilitates healing, and Archangel Michael, the angel of protection. All we have to do is ask them!

When faced with your own mortality, everything you thought was important to you changes. A life-threatening illness forces you to consider the fragility of life. I didn't think about the physical aspects of dying; I just knew I didn't want to leave my family—my husband and children. After experiencing the loss of my mom at a young age, I didn't want James and Leah to have that empty space in their lives. I wanted them to have their mom; I wanted to be there for the milestones and important moments in their lives. Besides, I hadn't finished mothering them yet!

Even after her death, my mom has always been there for me in spirit. It's not the same as having her human arms wrap around me, but I have no doubt that she is a presence in my life.

Our loved ones who have crossed over can visit us, guide us, and support us; sometimes we become aware of a subtle sign, and other times it's blatant. We just have to open our minds.

For instance, I'll share these thought-provoking moments:

It was a beautiful spring morning. I was in my bathroom drying my hair when suddenly I felt the strong presence of my mom. This was the third time I'd had this feeling over the last couple of days, and I wanted proof that it was not just my imagination. I spoke out loud, "Mom, if it really is you, I need a sign to let me know for sure." At that instant, the vision of a yellow flower popped into my mind. (She loved yellow flowers.) I persisted, "Okay, so sometime today I will see a yellow flower, and I will know that it really was you."

I finished drying my hair and went out to the kitchen. As I opened the refrigerator, my nephew, who had spent the night, burst through the door and handed me a yellow flower!

My mom's favorite sign to get my attention is feathers. I have found them in the oddest places. One morning when I was running, something appeared at eye level—one lone tiny white feather. Lone feathers have appeared inside the refrigerator, the washing machine, and the clothes dryer. Once, while I was vacuuming and mopping the kitchen floor, I asked the Universe to help with the sale of our house. After I finished cleaning, I glanced down to find a beautiful white feather there on the spotless tile by my feet. I knew my mom was there, watching over me. Another time, during a mid-morning walk, I was in a reflective mood and missing my mom. As I came upon a large grassy area, I couldn't help but notice one very large feather stuck in the soil, towering above the cut grass. One sleepless night I finally got out of bed. It was three o'clock in the morning, and I was sitting in front of my computer. Suddenly I felt I had company; I felt soothed, and I sensed my mom was there. When I clicked on a website, the word *daisy* stood out on the home page. The same word appeared on a second website. Daisy was my mother's name. Smiling to myself, I asked for confirmation, "Let me know it's you." Before going back to bed, I stopped in the kitchen for a drink of water. A magazine on the counter caught my eye. It was open to a page about flowers—daisies.

On the day my father's body succumbed to lung cancer, he was in hospice care at his home, and seven of his children were gathered around him. He was lying in bed, mostly silent. When he spoke, his words were weak. The photo of our mom he had asked for was placed next to him. As he went in and out of consciousness, he made the remark, "I am more there than I am here." I have no doubt he was communicating with angels in his last hours. His passing was very peaceful and sent tingles up my spine. In the moment before he took his last breath, he suddenly sat up with strength and energy we hadn't seen in a long time. He stretched his arms toward the sky and bellowed, "Thank you, Jesus!" In his last hours, we had each spent personal moments with him and said our good-byes. He hadn't replied when I told him I loved him, and it made me sad. At a later time, when my sisters and I were sorting his things, I noticed a calendar on his bedroom wall. Out of the blue, I felt a strong urge to look behind it. When I lifted the calendar, I saw a red heart made of yarn hanging beneath it. Inscribed in the middle were the words *I love you.*

Years ago I needed to buy ribbon for a craft project, and planned to stop by the fabric store, after picking up James and Leah from school. Having collected Leah as usual, I was surprised that we had to wait for James; his class had never been dismissed late before. Ten minutes later, we were in the car and on our way. As we arrived at the fabric store, we saw that an elderly lady had accidentally accelerated and crashed through the storefront; the car was halfway inside the fabric store and had mowed down everything in its path. We were told it had happened just ten minutes earlier. Had we not been delayed, we would have been walking into the store at that moment. How can I not believe in divine intervention?

On a particular February evening, I was sitting alone in my living room. My sister was struggling with a personal problem, and our family was extremely concerned about her well-being. Feeling distraught as I paced our living room, I begged out loud, "Please, God, please help her ... someone, please! At that instant a glass candleholder on the coffee table, which was suspended from a decorative hook, banged loudly against its metal support bracket. The sound startled me, and I froze. There was no breeze or air-conditioning that could have caused this. It was the anniversary of the day we had lost our mother. Maybe she was trying to let me know she had heard me. Someone was.

The signs are all around us, but they are easy to overlook, ignore, or dismiss as coincidence.

Throughout my life, I have taken risks and bent a few rules. Sometimes this attitude has served me well; sometimes not so much. But as Lucille Ball said, "I'd rather regret the things I've done than regret the things I haven't done."

Neale Donald Walsch's quote, "Life begins at the end of your comfort zone", is true on many levels.

We all encounter obstacles in our lives. With each challenge, we have choices to make. How am I going to deal with this? Am I going to be positive minded or negative? Thoughts and reactions to situations directly influence outcomes. Everything begins with a single thought.

Some may look at emotion as weakness, but emotion is energy. Emotion is cleansing and powerful. My tears gave me strength.

You can overcome and forge ahead, or you can succumb to misery and let it defeat you. We can choose which circumstances we accept in our lives and which ones we will eliminate.

It took me a long time to realize that meeting the "right guy" wasn't going to validate me; I needed to love myself. It is easy to feel inadequate and become deflated. Our inner critics talk too much, but one simple change in perspective can alter your mindset. Be kind to yourself. No one is flawless.

Our thoughts manifest our actions, and our actions manifest our reality. Set your intention. It is amazing what we can accomplish simply by setting the intent and acting on that belief. Worry less, because you have tremendous power—we all do! We just have to step into it. Don't give your power away.

I no longer say "my cancer." I do not accept it or take ownership of it. It is an invasive action within the body, and it is not welcome here.

I believe we are here to learn lessons. Everyone struggles. Some lives have sprinkles and showers; some have thunderstorms and hurricanes. What we consider to be a problem may actually be an opportunity to reach and grow. If life were all rainbows, what would we accomplish?

Years have passed since that dreadful day when I heard cancer had invaded my reality. The world looks different to me after breast cancer. I absorb moments that would have gone unnoticed, I cherish my loved ones, and I value my health. I've learned that when life hands you something you think you can't handle, you can. Just find your reason not to give up! Trust the journey.